MANUAL

FOR

STABLE SERGEANTS

1917

Fredonia Books
Amsterdam, The Netherlands

Manual for Stable Sergeants 1917

by
United States War Department

ISBN: 1-58963-612-0

Reprinted from the 1917 edition

Fredonia Books
Amsterdam, The Netherlands
http://www.fredoniabooks.com

WAR DEPARTMENT,
Washington, *June 14, 1917.*

The following Manual for Stable Sergeants, prepared at the Mounted Service School, Fort Riley, Kans., is published for the information and guidance of all concerned.

[2046213 A. G. O.]

BY ORDER OF THE SECRETARY OF WAR:

TASKER H. BLISS,
Major General, Acting Chief of Staff.

OFFICIAL:
H. P. McCAIN,
The Adjutant General.

3

AUTHORITIES CONSULTED.

Adams: A Text Book of Horseshoeing.
Bureau of Animal Industry: Special Report on Diseases of the Horse.
Chauveau: Comparative Anatomy of Domesticated Animals.
Dun: Veterinary Medicines, Their Actions and Uses.
Fitzwygram: Horses and Stables.
Flemming: Operative Veterinary Surgery.
Friedburger and Frohner: Pathology and Therapeutics of Domestic Animals.
Gay: Productive Horse Husbandry.
Goubaux and Barrier: The Exterior of the Horse.
Hayes: Points of the Horse.
Hayes: Veterinary Notes for Horse Owners.
Henry: Feeds and Feeding.
Hutyra and Marek: Pathology and Therapeutics of the Diseases of Domestic Animals.
Jordan: The Feeding of Animals.
Law: Veterinary Medicine.
Liautard: Manual of Veterinary Surgery.
Moller: Operative Veterinary Surgery.
Merillat: Veterinary Surgical Operations.
Neumann: Parasites and Parasitic Diseases of Domesticated Animals.
Quitman: Notes on Veterinary Materia Medica.
Sisson: A Text Book on Veterinary Anatomy.
Smith: Veterinary Hygiene.
Smith: A Manual of Veterinary Physiology.
Strangeway: Veterinary Anatomy.
Veterinary Department, English Army: Animal Management.
White: Principles and Practice of Veterinary Medicine.
Williams: Principles and Practice of Veterinary Medicine and Surgery.
Winslow: Materia Medica.
Woodhull: Military Hygiene.
Wyman: Diagnosis of Lameness in the Horse.

CONTENTS.

CONTENTS

LIST OF ILLUSTRATIONS.

9

MANUAL FOR STABLE SERGEANTS.

CHAPTER I.

ANATOMY AND PHYSIOLOGY.

1. Anatomy is the study of the parts and organs of the animal body with regard to their structure, shape, and position.

Physiology is a description of the functions or uses of these parts.

Anatomy embraces the study of the skeleton, the articulations, the muscles, the digestive system, the respiratory system, the urogenital system, the circulatory system, the lymphatic system, the nervous system, the eye, the ear, the skin.

The Skeleton.

2. The skeleton is the framework of hard structures of the body which supports the soft parts and vital organs. In the horse it consists of 205 bones, all of which are held together by means of ligaments and muscles in such a manner as to form a series of joints, levers, and pulleys. It is divided into *trunk* and *limbs*.

The trunk consists of the *skull, spinal column, ribs,* and *breast bone.*

The limbs, two anterior and two posterior, support the body and furnish the levers of propulsion.

3. Bones are classified as *long, flat, short,* and *irregular.*

Long bones are found in the limbs, where they support the weight of the body and act as levers of motion.

Flat bones help inclose cavities containing vital and important organs. In this manner the ribs and scapula protect the heart and lungs.

Short bones occur in the knee and hock and in the fetlock joints. Their function is that of breaking concussion.

Irregular bones are such as those of the spinal column and certain bones of the cranium. The bones of the cranium inclose and pro-

11

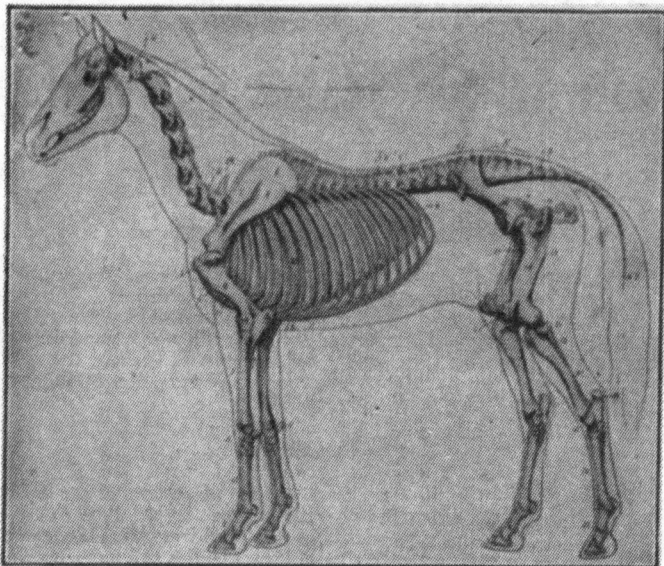

FIG 1.—Skeleton of horse, with outline of contour of body. *1. H.*, Atlas; *7.H.* seventh cervical vertebra; *1.R.*, first thoracic vertebra; *17.R.*, seventeenth thoracic vertebra; *1.L.*, first lumbar vertebra; *6 L.*, sixth lumbar vertebra; *K'*, sacrum; *1.S*, first coccygeal vertebra; *16 S.*, sixteenth coccygeal vertebra; *6.R.*, sixth rib; *6.K.*, costal cartilage; *18.R.*, last rib; 1, scapula; 1', cartilage of scapula; 2, spine of scapula; 4, humerus; 4' lateral epicondyle of humerus; 5, lateral tuberosity of humerus; 6, deltoid tuberosity; 7, shaft of ulna; 8, olecranon; 9, radius; 10, carpus; 11, accessory carpal bone; 12, metacarpus; 13, digit; 14, sternum; 14", xiphoid cartilage; 15, ilium; 16, 16', angles of ilium; 17, ischium; 18, femur (shaft); 19, trochanter major; 20, patella; 21, tibia (shaft); 21', lateral condyle of tibia; 23, fibula; 22, tarsus; 24, tuber calcis; 25, metatarsus; 26, digit; 27, trochanter minor of femur; 28, trochanter tertius of femur. (After Ellenberger-Baum, Anat. fur Kunstler) (From Sisson's Anatomy of the Domestic Animals; copyright, W. B. Saunders Co.)

tect the brain, while those of the spinal column inclose and protect the spinal cord.

All bones are covered with a tough membrane, the *periosteum*, except at their articular surfaces, where there is a layer of cartilage.

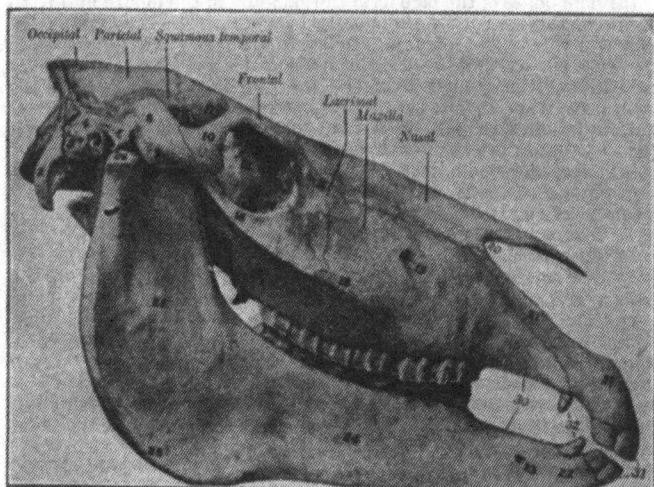

FIG. 2.—Skull of horse, right view. *1*, occipital condyle: *2*, paramastoid process; *3*, mastoid process; *4*, posterior process of squamous temporal bone; *5*, external acoustic process; *6*, zygomatic process of temporal bone; *7*, postglenoid process; *8*, glenoid cavity of squamous temporal bone, *9*, condyle of same; *10*, supraorbital process of frontal bone; *11*, temporal part of frontal bone; *12*, orbital part of frontal bone; *13*, fossa sacci lacrimalis; *14*, orbital surface of lacrimal bone; *15*, lacrimal tubercle; *16*, zygomatic process of malar bone; *17*, maxillary tuberosity; *18*, facial crest; *19*, infraorbital foramen; *20*, naso-maxillary notch; *21*, body of premaxilla; *21'*, nasal process of same; *22*, body of mandible, *23*, mental foramen; *24*, *25*, horizontal and vertical parts of ramus of mandible; *26*, condyle of mandible; *27*, coronoid process of mandible; *28*, angle of mandible; *29*, vascular impression; *30*, interalveolar margin; *31*, incisor teeth; *32*, canine teeth; *33*, hyoid bone (great cornu). (From Sisson's Anatomy of the Domestic Animals; copyright, W. B. Saunders.)

4. The skull (fig. 2) is the bony framework of the head. It consists of 34 irregularly-shaped flat bones, and is divided into two parts, the *cranium* and the *face*.

(*a*) The bones of the cranium inclose the brain, and, together with
the bones of the face, form the *orbital* and *nasal cavities*, in which are
situated the organs of *sight* and *smell*.

(*b*) The bones of the face form the skeleton of the mouth and nasal
cavities, and support the tongue and larynx. The most important
bones of this region are the *maxillae* (upper jaw) and the *mandible*
(lower jaw), each of which, on either side, presents six irregular
cavities for the reception of the *cheek* (molar) teeth. From the
orbital cavities forward the upper jaw gradually becomes narrower
and terminates in the *premaxilla*, which contains the six upper
incisor teeth; these six, with the corresponding teeth of the lower
jaw, help form the anterior boundary of the mouth.

(*c*) In each *maxilla*, just below the orbit, is an inclosed irregular-
shaped cavity known as the *maxillary sinus*. It connects with the
nasal cavity and contains the roots of the last three cheek teeth.

5. The teeth are 40 in number, and are of three kinds, viz:

(*a*) The *incisors*, 12 in number, are situated in the front part of the
mouth, 6 in the premaxilla and 6 in the anterior extremity of the
lower jaw.

(*b*) The *canines* (tushes), 4 in number, are situated in the *interdental space* just back of the incisors. In the *mare* these teeth are
usually very small or wanting entirely.

(*c*) The *cheek* teeth (molars), are 24 in number, and are situated in
the back part of the mouth, 6 above and 6 below on each side of each
jaw. The space between the incisors and molars is called the *interdental* space.

6. The spinal or vertebral column may be regarded as the basis
of the skeleton from which all other parts originate. It extends from
the base of the skull to the tip of the tail, and consists of a chain of
irregular bones called *vertebrae*, all solidly united by ligaments and
cartilage. According to their position in the column, they are divided into five regions, which are, naming them from front to rear,
the *cervical, thoracic, lumbar, sacral, and coccygeal*.

(*a*) In the *cervical* region there are 7 bones, which form the framework of the neck, the first being called the *atlas* and the second the
axis, the remaining 5 having no special names.

(*b*) The *thoracic vertebrae* are 18 in number. They furnish attachment for the upper ends of the ribs, and their superior spines, from
the second to the eighth, inclusive, form the framework of the
withers.

(c) The *lumbar* region consists of six bones forming the skeleton of the loins.

(d) In the *sacral* region there are five segments which become united to form a single bone, the *sacrum.*

(e) The *coccygeal vertebrae* are the last of the series. They number from 13 to 20 and form the skeleton of the tail.

(f) Throughout the length of this bony chain from the atlas to the fourth coccygeal vertebra, inclusive, is a tubular passage called the *spinal canal,* which is continuous with the cranium and which contains the spinal cord.

7. The bony thorax (chest) is a large cavity formed by the thoracic vertebrae above, the ribs on the sides and the *sternum* (breast bone) below. It contains the lungs, the heart, some large blood vessels and nerves, and a part of the trachea and the esophagus.

8. The ribs are 18 on each side, and are attached above to the thoracic vertebrae. Below, the first eight are attached to the sternum by means of cartilage, and are called *true* or *sternal* ribs. The remaining 10 are attached indirectly to the sternum and are called *false* or *asternal* ribs.

9. The bones of the fore limb, named from above downward, are the *scapula, humerus, radius,* and *ulna;* the *carpus* (knee) consisting of seven or eight small bones; the large *metacarpal* (cannon) bone; two small *metacarpal* (splint) bones; the *first phalanx* (long pastern bone); the *second phalanx* (short pastern bone); the *third phalanx* (coffin bone); two *proximal sesamoids,* and the *distal sesamoid* or *navicular* bone.

10. The bones of the hind limb, named from above downward, are the *os coxae* (hip bone), *femur* (thigh), *tibia, fibula,* and *patella* (stifle); the *tarsus* (hock), consisting of six or seven small bones; the *large metatarsal* (cannon bone); the two *small metatarsals* (splint bones); the *first phalanx* (long pastern bone); the *second phalanx* (short pastern bone); the *third phalanx* (coffin bone); two *proximal sesamoids,* and the *distal sesamoid* or navicular bone.

11. The os coxae (hip bone) consists of three parts, the *ilium ischium,* and *pubis,* all of which meet and unite to form a large cup-shaped cavity for articulation with the head of the femur. The right and left hip bones are connected above with the sacrum and below they are united with each other to form the *floor* of the *pelvic* cavity. This bony arch, together with the first three coccygeal vertebrae, is called the *pelvis* and forms the framework of the hips and croup.

The Articulations.

12. An articulation (joint) is the union of two or more bones or cartilages by strong fibrous bands called *ligaments*.

Joints are of three types—*immovable, slightly movable,* and *freely movable*.

(a) In movable joints the contact surfaces of the bones are covered with a thin, smooth layer of *articular cartilage*, the latter being lubricated with *synovia* or joint oil

13. Synovia is a thin oil-like fluid secreted by the *synovial membrane*. It is confined within and protected by the *joint capsule*, which completely surrounds the joint.

14. Ligaments, with the exception of the *ligamentum nuchae* (neck ligament), are composed of inelastic white fibrous tissue which bind the bones together.

15. Ligaments which hold the bones in position are known as *binding ligaments*. They are placed just outside the joint capsule with which they are closely related.

16. The suspensory ligament (figs. 5, 6, 7) is a long, wide band of white fibrous tissue, originating on the back part of the lower bones of the knee (hock bones in the hind leg) and the upper end of the cannon bone. It then passes downward between the splint bones and divides near the lower end of the cannon into two branches, which are attached one to each sesamoid bone. From these bones the branches pass downward and forward, one on the inner and one on the outer side of the long pastern bone, to become attached to the tendon of the muscle which extends the foot. Its function is to brace the fetlock joint and support a large portion of the body weight.

17. The ligamentum nuchae (neck ligament) is composed of yellow elastic tissue, and extends from the withers forward, above the cervical vertebræ, to become attached to the top of the skull. It supports the head and neck.

18. The plantar ligament is located on the outer posterior border of the hock. It is one of the important binding ligaments of the hock joint.

19. The joints of the fore limb, named from above downward, are the *shoulder joint*, formed by the *scapula* and *humerus;* the *elbow joint*, formed by the *humerus, radius,* and *ulna;* the *carpal* (knee) *joint*, formed by the *radius*, the bones of the *carpus*, and the large and the two small *metacarpal* bones; the *fetlock joint*, formed by the large *metacarpal* bone, the *proximal sesamoids*, and the *first phalanx;* the *pastern joint*, formed by the *first* and *second phalanges;* and the *coffin joint*, formed by the *second* and *third phalanges* and the *navicular bone*

20. The joints of the hind limb, named from above downward, are the *sacro-iliac joint;* formed by the *sacrum* and *ilium;* the *hip joint*, formed by the *hip bone* and the *femur;* the *stifle joint*, formed by the *femur*, the *patella*, and *tibia*; the *tarsal* (hock) *joint*, formed by the *tibia*, the *bones* of the *hock*, and the large and small *metatarsal* bones. The joints below the hock are named and formed the same as in the fore limb.

THE MUSCLES.

21. Muscles are the active organs of motion and are classified as *voluntary* and *involuntary*. Voluntary muscles are those under direct control of the will, as the muscles of the leg and tail. Involuntary muscles are those not under direct control of the will, as the heart and the muscles of the intestines. The voluntary muscles form about 45 per cent of the weight of the body.

22. Muscles are composed of a *contractile* part, which is red in color and forms the flesh; and a *tendinous* part, which is usually attached to the bones but may be attached to other muscles. *Tendons* are similar in structure to ligaments, being composed of white inelastic fibers. Their function is to transmit to the point of attachment the power generated by the contraction of the fleshy portion of the muscle.

23. With regard to their form muscles are classified as *long*, *wide*, and *short*. Wide muscles surround the body cavities. Short muscles are found near the joints and irregular shaped bones. Long muscles are found in the limbs, in the neck, and along the back.

24. A muscle is an *extensor* when its action is to extend, or straighten, a joint; it is a *flexor* when its action is to flex, or bend, a joint. The following paragraphs (25 and 26) contain a brief description of a few important extensors and flexors of the limbs.

25. Muscles of the fore limb (fig. 5, 6).

(*a*) The *common digital extensor* (common extensor of the foot) (fig. 5c). This is the principal extensor of the fore leg and foot. It originates at the lower extremity of the *humerus*, and its fleshy portion continues to the lower end of the *radius*, at which point it becomes tendinous, passes downward over the knee, and continues along the front of the cannon to become attached to the upper and front part of the *third phalanx*.

Action.—To *extend* the joints of the foot and knee.

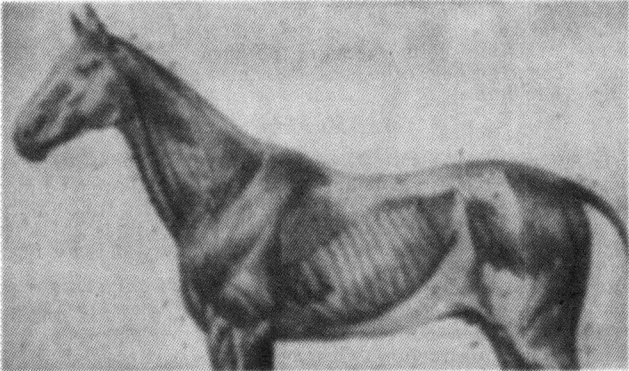

FIG. 3.—Superficial muscles of horse. The cutaneous muscle, except the cervical part, has been removed. *a*, Trapezius cervicalis; *a'*, trapezius thoracalis; *c, c*, brachiocephalicus; *d*, sterno-cephalicus; *e*, deltoid; *f*, long head of triceps, *f'*, lateral head of triceps; *g*, anterior superficial pectoral; *h*, posterior deep pectoral; *h'*, anterior deep pectoral; *i*, serratus thoracis; *i'*, serratus cervicis, *k*, latissimus dorsi; *l*, obliquus abdominis externus; *l'*, aponeurosis of *l*; *m*, serratus dorsalis; *m'*, lumbo-dorsal fascia; *o*, tensor fasciae latae; *o'*, fascia lata; *o''*, gluteus superficialis; *p'*, gluteal fascia; *q, q', q''*, biceps femoris; *r*, semitendinosus; *s*, sacro-coccygeus dorsalis; *t*, sacro-coccygeus lateralis; *u*, coccygeus; *v*, cervical cutaneous muscle; *w*, splenius; *x*, rhomboideus; *y*, tendon of longissimus capitis et atlantis and brachiocephalicus; *z*, supraspinatus; *z'*, external intercostal; ✕, wing of atlas; *2*, spine of scapula; *4'*, lateral epicondyle of humerus; *6*, deltoid tuberosity; *8*, olecranon; *16*, tuber coxae; *20*, patella; *21'*, lateral condyle of tibia. (After Ellenberger-Baum, Anat. fur Kunstler) (From Sisson's Anatomy of the Domestic Animals; Copyright, W. B. Saunders Co.)

(*b*) The *superficial digital flexor* (superficial flexor of the foot) (fig. 6). This muscle originates from the lower and inner part of the *humerus*. It passes down the back part of the leg, becoming tendinous just above the knee; from the knee it passes downward to the fetlock where it expands and forms a ring for the passage of the deep flexor tendon.   At the lower end of the first phalanx the tendon divides into two branches which become attached one on either side of the upper end of the *second phalanx*.   The tendon of this

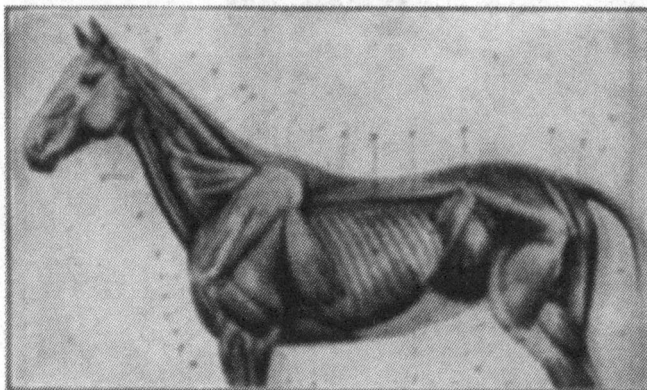

FIG. 4.—Deeper muscles of horse. *d*, Sterno-cephalicus; *f*, long head of triceps; *f'* lateral head of triceps; *g*, anterior superficial pectoral; *h*, posterior deep pectoral *h'*, anterior deep pectoral, *ı*, serratus thoracis; *i'*, serratus cervicis; *l*, obliquus abdominis externus, and *l'*, its aponeurosis, the posterior part of which has been removed; *m*, serratus dorsalis posterior; *p*, gluteus medius; *r*, semitendinosus ; *s*, sacro-coccygeus dorsalis; *t*, sacro-coccygeus lateralis; *u*, coccygeus; *v'*, biceps brachii; *x*, rhomboideus; *y*, *y'*, longissimus capitis et altantis; *c*, supraspinatus; *z'*, infraspinatus; *1'*, cartilage of scapula; *2*, spine of scapula; *5*, lateral tuberosity of humerus; *6*, deltoid tuberosity; *8*, olecranon; *16*, tuber coxae; *19*, trochanter major; *20*, patella; *21'*, lateral condyle of tibia; *26*, transverse processes of cervical vertebrae; *27*, parotido-auricularis; *28*, vastus lateralis; *28'*, rectus femoris; *28''*, trochanter tertius; *29*, semimembranosus; *30*, gastrocnemius; *31*, sacro-sciatic ligament; *32*, omo-hyoideus; *33*, complexus; *34*, rectus capitis ventralis major; *35*, spinalis dorsi, *36*, longissimus dorsi, *37*, longissimus costarum; *38*, teres minor; *39*, brachialis, *40*, external intercostal, *41*, obliquus abdominis internus; *42*, iliacus; *43*, transversus abdominis. (After Ellenberger-Baum, Anat. fur Künstler.) (From Sisson's Anatomy of the Domestic Animals; copyright, W. B. Saunders Co)

muscle lies behind the cannon, immediately under the skin, and covers the deep flexor tendon.

Action.—To flex the knee, fetlock, and pastern.

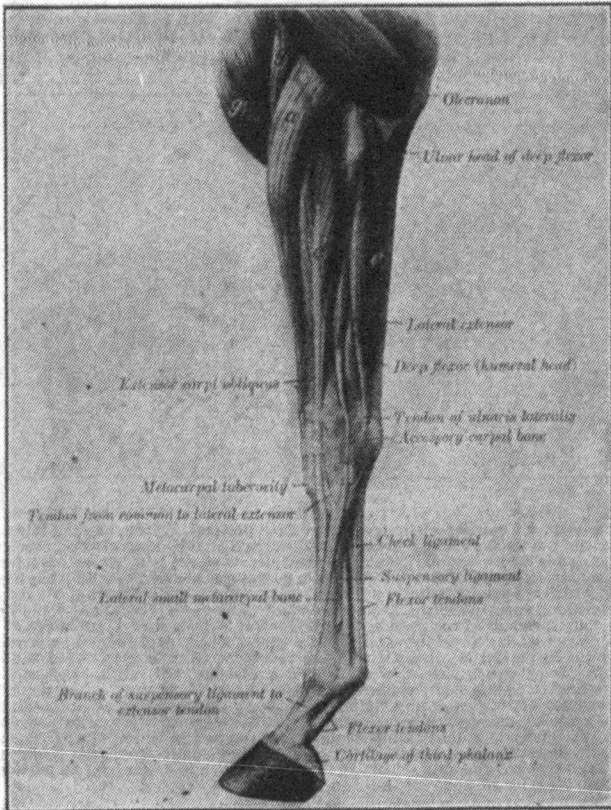

FIG. 5.—Muscles of left thoracic limb of horse from elbow downward, lateral
view. a, Extensor carpi radialis; g, brachialis; g', anterior superficial pectoral;
c, common digital extensor; e, ulnaris lateralis. (After Ellenberger-Baum,
Anat. für Kunstler.) (From Sisson's Anatomy of the Domestic Animals;
copyright, W. B. Saunders Co.)

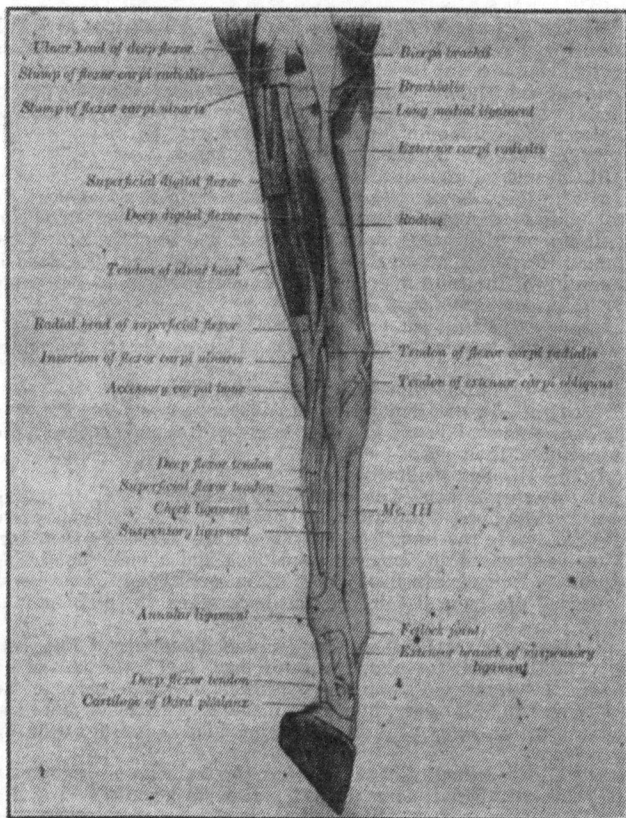

FIG. 6.—Muscles of left thoracic limb of horse, from elbow downward, medial
\view. Parts of superficial muscles have been removed, carpal canal opened
up, and flexor tendons drawn backward. (From Sisson's Anatomy of the
Domestic Animals; copyright, W. B. Saunders Co.)

(c) The *deep digital flexor* (deep flexor of the foot) (fig. 6). This muscle originates with the superficial digital flexor. Its tendinous portion begins at the knee, passes down the leg between the cannon bone and the tendon of the superficial flexor, over the back part of the fetlock, through the ring formed by the superficial tendon, and is attached to the under surface of the *third phalanx*.

Action.—To *flex* the knee and all joints below it.

26. Muscles of the hind limb (fig. 7).

(a) The *long digital extensor* (long extensor of the foot) (fig. 7). This muscle originates from the lower and front part of the femur; its fleshy portion passes downward along the front surface of the tibia to the hock, where it becomes tendinous; from the hock it passes down the front of the leg to become attached to the upper and front part of the *third phalanx*.

Action.—To *extend* the foot and flex the hock.

(b) *Tibialis anterior* (anterior tibial). This muscle lies in front of the tibia.

Origin.—From the front and outer border of the tibia.

Insertion.—By two tendons, one to the upper and front part of the *large metatarsal* bone; the other to one of the small bones on the inner side of the hock.

Action.—To flex the hock joint.

(c) *Peroneus tertius.*—This is a strong tendinous cord, extending from the lower end of the front part of the *femur* to the hock where it terminates in two branches—a large one inserted in the front part of the upper end of the *large metatarsal bone*, and a small one passing outward to become attached to one of the small bones of the hock.

Action.—Mechanically to flex the hock when the stifle joint is flexed.

(d) The *superficial digital flexor* (superficial flexor of the foot) (fig. 7) of the hind leg originates at the back and lower part of the *femur*. It extends downward back of the tibia to the point of the hock over which it passes; thence down the back of the leg to be disposed of in the same manner as the superficial digital flexor of the front leg.

Action.—To extend the hock and flex the fetlock and pastern.

(e) The *deep digital flexor* (deep flexor of the foot) (fig. 7) of the hind leg originates from the upper and back part of the *tibia*, near the lower third of which it becomes tendinous and passes downward over the inner and back side of the hock to become attached to the *third phalanx* in the same manner as the deep flexor of the fore leg.

Action.—To extend the hock and flex the joints below it.

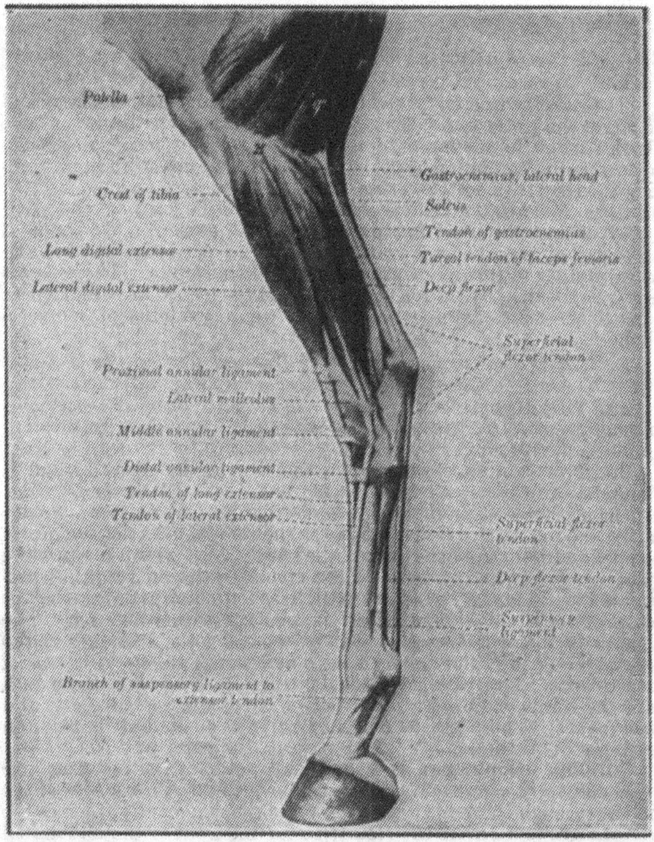
Patella
Crest of tibia
Long digital extensor
Lateral digital extensor
Gastrocnemius, lateral head
Soleus
Tendon of gastrocnemius
Tarsal tendon of biceps femoris
Deep flexor
Superficial flexor tendon
Proximal annular ligament
Lateral malleolus
Middle annular ligament
Distal annular ligament
Tendon of long extensor
Tendon of lateral extensor
Superficial flexor tendon
Deep flexor tendon
Branch of suspensory ligament to

FIG. 7. Muscles of lower part of thigh, leg, and foot of horse, lateral view. *o′*, Fascia lata; *q*, *q′*, *q″*, biceps femoris; *r*, semitendinosus; *21′*, lateral condyle of tibia. The extensor brevis is visible in the angle between the long and lateral extensor tendons, but by an oversight it is not marked (After Ellenberger-Baum, Anat. fur Kunstler) (From Sisson's Anatomy of the Domestic Animals; copyright, W. B. Saunders Co.)

(*f*) *Gastrocnemius* (fig. 7). This muscle originates at the lower and back of the *femur* and is attached to the point of the hock. At the back part of the leg the tendon of this muscle becomes closely associated with the tendon of the superficial digital flexor, the two forming the tendon of *achilles*, or *hamstring*.

Action.—To extend the hock and flex the stifle joint

27. Synovial membranes (synovial bursæ and synovial sheaths) of tendons and muscles (figs. 8, 9, 10, 11) are thin-walled sacs, similar to the synovial membranes of the joints. They secrete synovia for the prevention of friction and are placed at points where one structure moves upon another, as where a tendon plays over a bone.

THE DIGESTIVE SYSTEM.

28. The digestive organs are the *mouth, pharynx, esophagus, stomach, small intestine, large intestine, and anus;* all lined with mucous membrane.

29. The mouth extends from the lips to the pharynx and is bounded on the sides by the cheeks and above by the *hard palate.* Its floor is formed by the tongue and other muscular tissue. Separating the mouth from the pharynx is the *soft palate*, a fleshy curtain suspended from the back part of the hard palate, which permits the passage of food and water from the mouth to the pharynx but prevents its passage in the opposite direction. The *lips* are the organs of *prehension* (picking up) and possess the sense of touch. The *tongue* is a muscular organ, situated between the branches of the lower jaw. It is the organ of taste and assists in the processes of mastication, insalivation, and swallowing. Opening into the mouth are the ducts of the *salivary glands*—the *parotid, submaxillary,* and *sublingual*. These glands are six in number, located in pairs on either side of the mouth. The *pharynx*, see paragraph 50.

30. The esophagus is a muscular tube extending from the pharynx to the stomach. It passes down the lower left side of the neck, through the middle portion of the thoracic cavity, pierces the diaphragm and enters the stomach near the front of the abdominal cavity.

31. The stomach (fig. 13) is a hollow, pear-shaped organ, situated in the anterior and left side of the abdominal cavity, behind the liver. Its internal, or mucous, coat is divided into a right and a

Fig. 8.—Synovial sheaths and bursæ of distal part of right fore limb of horse, medial view. The synovial sheaths (colored yellow) and the joint capsules (colored pink) are injected. a, Sheath of extensor carpi obliquus; b, sheath of flexor carpi radialis; c, carpal sheath; d, d', d", d''', digital sheath; e, bursa under common extensor tendon; f, capsule of fetlock joint; 1, extensor carpi radialis; 2, tendon of extensor carpi obliquus; 3, flexor carpi radialis; 4, flexor carpi ulnaris; 5, superficial flexor tendon; 6, deep flexor tendon; 7, suspensory ligament; 8, small metacarpal bone; 9, large metacarpal bone; 10, volar annular ligament of fetlock; 11, proximal digital annular ligament; 12, radius; 13, radiocarpal joint; 14, fetlock joint; 15, cartilage of third phalanx; 16, band from first phalanx to cartilage. (After Ellenberger, in Leisering's Atlas) (From Sisson's Anatomy of the Domestic Animals; copyright, W. B. Saunders Co)

Fig. 9.—Synovial sheaths and bursæ of distal part of right fore limb of horse, lateral view. The synovial sheaths (colored yellow) and the joint capsules (colored ink) are injected. a, Sheath of extensor carpi radialis; b, sheath of common extensor; c, sheath of lateral extensor; d, sheath of outer tendon of ulnaris lateralis; e, e', carpal sheath; f, f', f", digital sheath; g, bursa under common extensor tendon; h, bursa under lateral extensor tendon; i, capsule of fetlock joint; 1, extensor carpi radialis; 2, common digital extensor; 3, lateral digital extensor; 4, ulnaris lateralis; 4', 4", tendons of 4; 5, superficial flexor tendon; 6, deep flexor tendon; 7, suspensory ligament; 8, lateral metacarpal bone; 9, large metacarpal bone; 10, volar annular ligament of fetlock; 11, digital annular ligament; 12, fetlock joint; 13, cartilage of third phalanx; 14, band from first phalanx to cartilage. (After Ellenberger, in Leisering's Atlas.) (From Sisson's Anatomy of the Domestic Animals; copyright, W. B. Saunders Co.)

Fig 10.—Injected synovial sheaths and bursæ of tarsal region of horse, medial view. a, Synovial sheath of peroneus tertius and tibialis anterior; b, bursa under medial (cunean) tendon of tibialis anterior; c, synovial sheath of flexor longus; d, tarsal sheath of deep flexor; e, e', bursa under superficial flexor tendon; f, f', tibio-tarsal joint capsule; 1, long extensor; 2, tibialis anterior; 2', medial (cunean) tendon of 2; 3, flexor longus; 4, deep digital flexor; 5, superficial flexor tendon; 6, gastrocnemius tendon; 7, tibia; 8, tarsus; 9, tuber calcis; 10, large metatarsal bone; 11, medial small metatarsal bone; 12, 12', fascial bands. (After Ellenberger, in Leisering's Atlas) (From Sisson's Anatomy of the Domestic Animals; copyright, W. B. Saunders Co.)

Fig. 11.—Injected synovial sheaths and bursæ of tarsal region of horse, lateral view. a, Synovial sheath of long digital extensor; b, synovial sheath of lateral digital extensor; c, c', bursa under superficial flexor tendon; d, capsule of hock joint; 1, long extensor; 2, lateral extensor; 3, 3, 3, annular ligaments; 4, deep digital flexor; 5, tendon of gastrocnemius; 6, superficial flexor tendon; 7, tibia; 8, tarsus; 9, tuber calcis; 10, metatarsus. (After Ellenberger, in Leisering's Atlas.) (From Sisson's Anatomy of the Domestic Animals; copyright, W. B. Saunders Co.)

24a

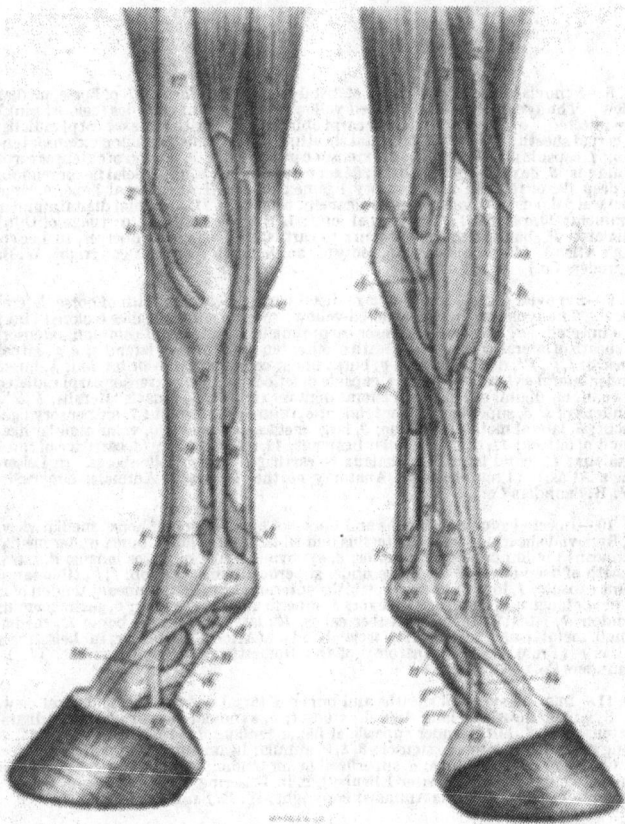

Fig. 8.   Fig. 9.

(See Page 29.)

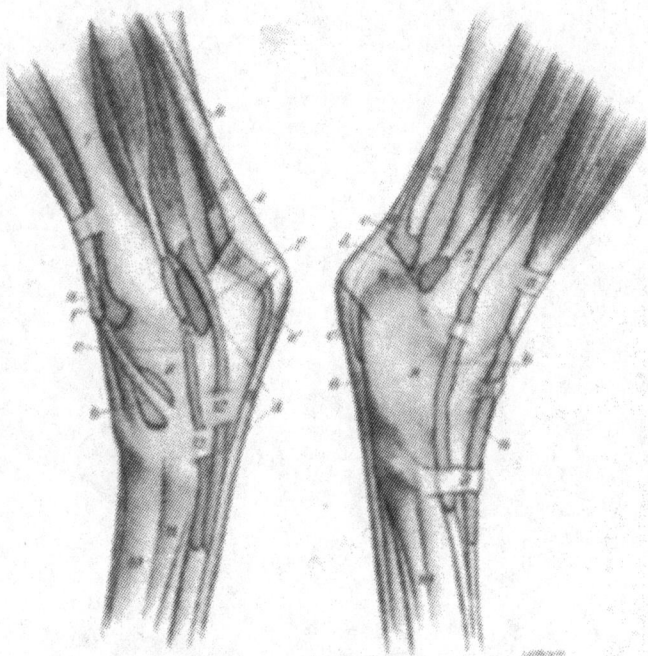

left portion. The left, or *cuticular*, portion has a hard, yellowish white surface which is continuous with the lining of the esophagus. The right, *villous*, or true digestive portion is reddish in color, vascular, and contains the *peptic glands* which secrete the *gastric juice*.

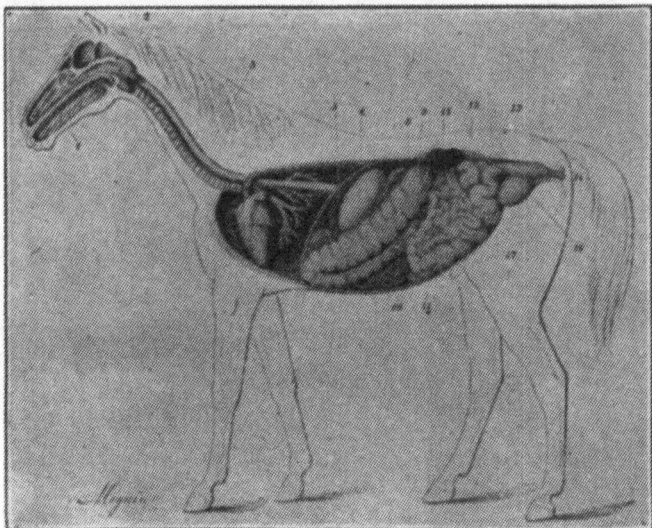

FIG. 12.—Digestive apparatus. 1, mouth; 2, pharynx; 3, esophagus; 4, diaphragm; 5, liver; 6, stomach (left sac); 8, liver, upper extremity; 9, large colon; 10, cæcum; 11, small intestines; 12, floating colon; 13, rectum, 14, anus; 15, left kidney and its ureter; 16, bladder; 17, urethra.

The capacity of the horse's stomach (from 3 to 4 gallons) is small in proportion to the size of the animal.

32. The small intestine extends from the stomach to the large intestine. It is about 70 feet long and from one to two inches in diameter.

33. The large intestine is about 22 feet long and varies in diameter. It consists of four parts, the *cæcum, great colon, small colon,* and *rectum.*

34. The mucous membrane of the intestines is covered with minute projections called *villi,* which absorb the nutriment of the

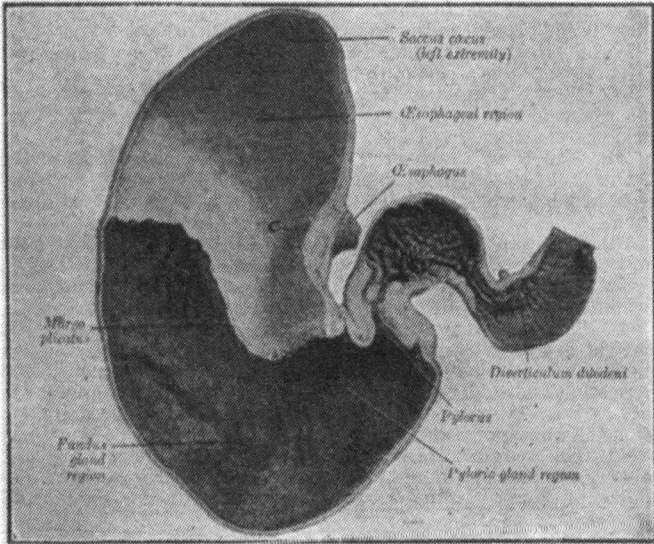

FIG. 13.—Frontal section of stomach and first part of duodenum of horse. *C,* Cardiac orifice. Photograph of specimen fixed *in situ.* (From Sisson's Anatomy of the Domestic Animals; copyright, W. B. Saunders Co.)

food after it has been prepared by digestion. The mucous membrane also contains small glands which pour their secretions into the intestines. These glands and villi are more numerous in the small intestine than in the large.

35. The anus is a muscular ring forming the posterior opening of the alimentary canal. It appears as a round projection below the root of the tail.

36. The stomach and intestines are suspended in the abdominal cavity by strong, fibrous bands, *the mesentery,* which are attached above to the lower surface of the muscle below the spinal column. Accompanying these fibrous bands are blood vessels, lymphatic vessels and glands, and nerves. Inclosing the intestines and lining the abdominal cavity is a serous membrane called the *peritoneum.* The mesentery is a part of the peritoneum.

37. In the abdominal cavity are three large glands, the *liver, pancreas,* and *spleen.* The spleen is a ductless gland. The liver and the pancreas are part of the digestive system.

38. The liver lies behind the diaphragm and in front of the stomach. It weighs from 10 to 12 pounds. Its function is to secrete *bile,* which is poured into the small intestines, where it aids digestion.

39. The pancreas is situated behind the stomach and in front of the kidneys, in the upper portion of the abdominal cavity. It weighs about 17 ounces. Its function is to secrete *pancreatic fluid,* which is poured into the small intestine, to aid in digestion.

40. The spleen is attached to the left side of the stomach. It is reddish gray in color and weighs from 2 to 3 pounds. Its function is not definitely known, but it is supposed to be concerned in the formation and destruction of blood corpuscles. It also appears to act as a reservoir for the extra supply of blood required by the stomach during digestion.

41. The abdominal cavity is inclosed by the muscles of the back above, the abdominal muscles on the sides and below, and the diaphragm in front. In the rear it is continuous with the *pelvic cavity.*

PHYSIOLOGY OF DIGESTION.

42. The function of the digestive organs as a whole is to take in the food, digest it, absorb the nutriment, and discharge the waste material from the body. The various steps are as follows:

43. Food is taken into the mouth by the lips, *prehension,* and is there ground up by the teeth, *mastication,* and mixed with saliva, *insalivation. Saliva,* which is secreted by the salivary glands, moistens the food and acts chemically upon certain parts. The tongue determines the taste of the food and by its muscular action assists in insalivation. From the mouth the food is carried back by the tongue to the pharynx. As soon as it reaches the pharynx the act of swallowing becomes involuntary and is completed by the pharynx and esophagus.

44. When the food reaches the stomach it is subjected to a mechanical rolling and mixing in the left side of the stomach (*maceration*). It gradually passes to the right side of the stomach, where it is acted upon by the gastric juice. It then passes into the small intestine and is called *chyme*.

45. In the small intestine, the chyme is acted on by the bile and pancreatic fluid and is then called *chyle*. The villi of the small intestines take up those parts of the food that have been rendered absorbable by digestion and the remainder is passed on to the cecum, which is the water reservoir. Here it is soaked and digestion continues slowly in the cecum and great colon. The digested parts of the food are absorbed here and the waste materials are passed on into the small colon. In the small colon the moisture is absorbed and the residue is formed into pellets of dung which are stored in the rectum, to be discharged at intervals through the anus (defecation).

THE RESPIRATORY SYSTEM.

46. The respiratory system consists of the *nostrils*, *nasal chambers*, *pharynx*, *larynx*, *trachea*, *bronchi*, and the *lungs*, all of which, except the air sacs, are lined with mucous membrane.

47. A mucous membrane is a thin layer of tissue lining all cavities and canals of the body which communicate with the external air.

48. Serous membranes are thin, glistening structures which line the cavities of the body and cover to a certain extent the organs therein contained. They secrete a fluid called *serous fluid* (serum) which moistens their surfaces and prevents friction. The synovial membranes, the peritoneum, and the plurae are serous membranes.

49. The nostrils are two oblong openings above the upper lip. They are the anterior openings of the nasal chambers.

50. The nasal chambers extend from the nostrils to the pharynx and occupy the bony canals above the mouth, from which they are separated by the hard palate. They are separated from each other by the cartilaginous *septum nasi*. Each chamber is divided into three passages by the *turbinated* bones.   The sense of smell is located at the back of the nasal chambers

51. The pharynx is an elongated cylindrical muscular cavity common to the respiratory and digestive tracts.   It lies just back of

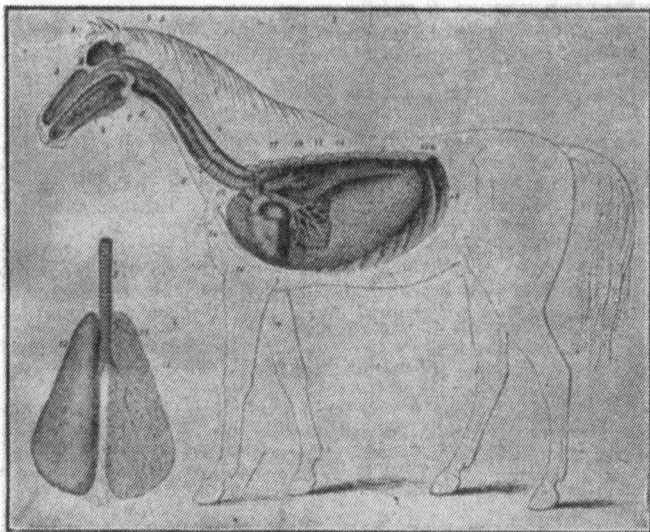

FIG. 14.—Respiratory apparatus.   3, Nasal chamber; 4, tongue; 5, pharynx; 6, larynx; 7, epiglottis, or potlid; 8, trachea, or windpipe, 9, Esophagus, or gullet; 10, section of left bronchus; 11, ramifications of the right bronchus; 12, right lung; 13, left lung, seen from above; 14, sternum, 15, ribs; 15a, section of the left ribs; 16, heart; 17, posterior aorta (cut off); 18, anterior aorta (cut off).

the mouth, above the larynx, and is continued backward by the esophagus.

52. The larynx is a muscular, cartilaginous box, situated in the back part of the maxillary space.   It has an anterior opening into the pharynx and a posterior one into the trachea, with which it is continuous. It gives passage to the air on its way to and from the lungs, and is the organ of voice. The anterior opening is guarded by a flexible cartilage called the *epiglottis*, which closes mechanically in the act of swallowing and prevents the passage of food or water into the larynx, trachea, and lungs.

53. **The trachea** is a flexible cylindrical tube, composed of from 40 to 50 incomplete cartilaginous rings, the number varying according to the length of the neck. It extends from the larynx to the base of the heart, where it divides into the *right* and *left bronchi*. These enter the lungs and subdivide into the *bronchial tubes*, the final subdivisions terminating in the air cells. The bronchi and bronchial tubes have cartilaginous plates in their walls to prevent their collapse. The *air cells* are minute sacs composed of a single layer of tissue cells and are surrounded by a network of capillaries.

54. **The lungs,** the essential organs of respiration, are two light, spongy organs of conical shape, situated in the thoracic cavity, one on either side. They are composed of elastic fibrous tissue and contain *bronchial tubes, air cells, blood vessels, lymphatic vessels,* and *nerves.*

55. **The thoracic cavity** is inclosed by the thoracic vertebrae, ribs, sternum, the muscles between the ribs (intercostal muscles), and the diaphragm. It contains the lungs, heart, large blood vessels, lymph vessels, nerves, the posterior portion of the trachea, the bronchi and a portion of the esophagus. The thoracic cavity is lined by two serous sacs, the right and left *pleurae*.

56. **The diaphragm** is a muscular and tendinous partition forming the posterior wall of the thoracic cavity and separating it from the abdomen.

57. **Respiration** consists of two acts; *inspiration*, the drawing of the air into the lungs; and *expiration*, the expulsion of the air from the lungs. These acts are involuntary and are controlled by the nervous system. When the horse is at rest respiration occurs about 12 times per minute. The amount of air taken in at each inspiration is about 250 cubic inches, the same amount being expelled at each expiration.

The Urogenital System.

58. The urinary organs are the *kidneys, ureters, bladder,* and *urethra.*

59. The kidneys are two glands situated one on either side of the spinal column immediately below the lumbar vertebrae. Their function is to separate waste material (urine) from the blood.

60. The ureters are two fibrous tubes conveying the urine from the kidneys to the bladder.

61. The bladder is a muscular sac in which the urine is stored until discharged from the body.

62. The urethra is a mucous tube which extends from the bladder to the head of the penis, in the male. In the female it extends from the bladder to the floor of the vagina, about 3 inches from the external opening.

63. The urine is a yellowish fluid composed of water, various salts, and waste materials from the body. The normal amount secreted is from 3 to 6 quarts in 24 hours. The color and quantity are variable, due to variations in food, work, and the temperature of the air.

64. The principal male generative organs are the *testicles* and *penis.*

65. The female generative organs are the *ovaries, fallopian tubes, uterus, vagina,* and *vulva.*

The Circulatory System.

66. The circulatory system consists of the *heart, arteries, capillaries, veins,* and the *blood.*

67. The heart (fig. 16) is a hollow organ, made up of involuntary muscles. It is situated in the middle and left side of the thoracic cavity, between the lungs, and is inclosed in a serous sac called the *pericardium.* In shape it is a blunt cone with the base upward and it weighs about 6½ pounds. It is divided into two parts, *right* and *left,* by a longitudinal muscular wall, or *septum.* Each part is divided into two cavities, the *atrium* above and the *ventricle* below. On each side the atrium and the ventricle communicate by openings which are guarded by valves to prevent the back flow of blood, but there is no communication between the two sides. The function of the heart is to maintain the circulation by continually pumping the blood through the arteries as it receives it from the veins.

68. Arteries are strong thick-walled tubes which carry the blood from the heart to all parts of the body. They give off branches and subdivide until they terminate in the capillaries.

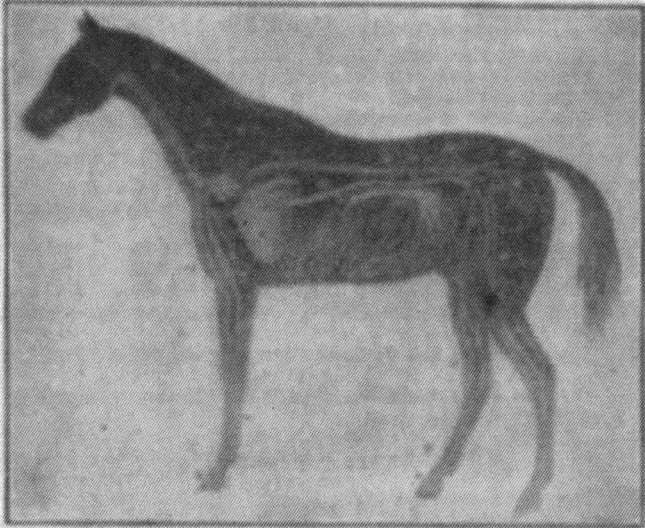

FIG. 15.—Circulatory apparatus. 1, Heart (right ventricle); 2, heart (left ventricle) 3, heart (left auricle); 3a, heart (right auricle); 4, pulmonary arteries (cut off); 5, pulmonary veins (cut off); 6, anterior aorta; 7, common carotid artery; 9, left brachial artery; 13, humeral artery; 14, radial artery; 15, metacarpal artery; 16; digital artery; 17, posterior aorta; 18, branches distributed to the stomach, spleen; pancreas, etc.; 19, branches distributed to the intestines, 20, branch to the kidneys; 22, posterior vena cava; 24, external iliac artery, 25, internal iliac artery; 27, femoral artery; 28, posterior tibial artery; 29, metatarsal artery; 30, venous network of the foot, 33, jugular vein, 34, anterior vena cava.

69. Capillaries are small, thin-walled vessels that are just large enough to permit the passage of the blood corpuscles In these vessels occurs the exchange of substances between the blood and the tissues, the tissues being supplied with oxygen and nutritious

material, the blood receiving waste in the form of carbonic acid gas.
An exception to this process is found in the capillaries surrounding
the air cells of the lungs, where the blood gives off carbonic acid gas
and receives oxygen. The capillaries form a close network in all
the tissues of the body, but are invisible to the naked eye.

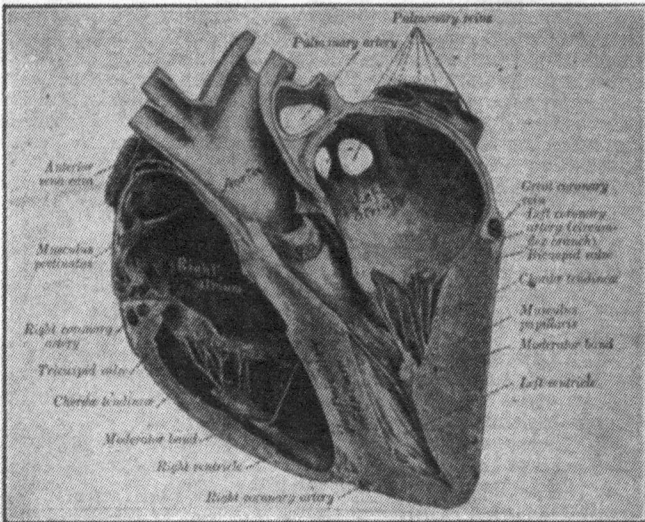

FIG. 16.—Section of heart of horse. Specimen hardened *in situ* and cut nearly at
right angles to the ventricular septum. The left ventricle is contracted, but not
ad maximum. V. a., Segment of aortic valve. (From Sisson's Anatomy of the
Domestic Animals, copyright, W. B. Saunders Co.)

70. **Veins** are the vessels that return the blood to the heart.
They begin at the capillaries and by uniting form larger veins which
finally empty into the atria. Veins differ from arteries in that
their walls are thinner and less firm, and by their having valves
which prevent the blood flowing backward within them. Veins

accompany arteries, as a rule, and bear the same names; among
exceptions to this rule may be noted the *anterior* and *posterior vena
cava* and the *jugular veins*. The circulation through the veins is
assisted by the contraction of the muscles during movement and
respiration.

71. **The blood** is a fluid which carries oxygen and nutritive
material to all the tissues of the body and, together with the lymph,
carries the waste material to the excretory organs. It is an opaque,
thickish fluid with a salty taste. Its color varies, being a *bright red*
or *scarlet* in the arteries and a *dark purple* in the veins, except in the
pulmonary artery, which carries purple or venous blood, and the
pulmonary veins, which carry red or arterial blood. It forms a
clot when the blood vessels are ruptured and the blood is exposed
to the air or tissues.

72. **Blood** is composed of *serum* and *red* and *white corpuscles*. The
serum is a thin, *yellowish* fluid in which the corpuscles float. It contains the soluble nutrient material from the food.

73. **The red corpuscles** carry *oxygen* to the tissues and *carbonic
acid gas* away from them. When they are charged with oxygen they
give the scarlet color to the blood, and the purple color when charged
with carbonic acid gas. The red corpuscles are formed in the bone
marrow.

74. **The white corpuscles** repair and assist in replacing worn out,
diseased or injured tissues. They also protect the tissues by destroying the germs which produce disease. They are formed in the
lymphatic glands and the spleen.

75. There are two divisions of the circulation, the *pulmonary*
and the *systemic*.

(*a*) The *pulmonary circulation* takes the blood from the heart to
the lungs and back to the heart. The impure blood from the whole of
the body enters the *right atrium* by the *anterior* and *posterior venae
cavae*; from the *right atrium* it passes to the *right ventricle*; from the
right ventricle it is pumped through the *pulmonary artery* to the *lungs*,
where it is *purified* by giving off *carbonic acid gas* and taking up *oxygen*. From the *lungs* the now purified blood is returned to the *heart*
through the *pulmonary veins* and emptied into the *left atrium*.

(*b*) The *systemic circulation*. From the *left atrium* the blood passes
into the *left ventricle*, thence into the *aorta* to be pumped to *all parts*
of the body, being distributed by means of *arteries* and *capillaries;*
from the *capillaries* it is collected by *veins* and brought back to the

right atrium through the *anterior* and *posterior venae cavae* to be again sent to the lungs for purification.

76. The aorta is the beginning of the arterial system. It is given off at the base of the *left ventricle* and divides into *thoracic* and *abdominal* parts.

(*a*) The *thoracic aorta* passes forward and divides into branches which supply the front part of the *thorax*, the *front limbs*, the *neck*, and the *head*.

(*b*) The *abdominal aorta* passes upward and backward, below the spinal column, to the last lumbar vertebrae where it divides into four branches which are distributed to the *hind quarters* and *posterior limbs*. Between its origin at the base of the left ventricle and its termination in the lumbar region it gives off branches to the *muscles* of the *ribs*, the *lungs* (for their nourishment), *liver stomach*, *spleen*, *pancreas*, *intestines*, *kidneys*, and *muscles* of the *loins*.

77. (*a*) The *anterior vena cava*, a large, short vein, returns the blood from the parts supplied by the thoracic aorta. It is located in the front part of the thorax and empties its blood into the *right atrium*.

(*b*) The *posterior vena cava*, the *largest* and *longest* vein in the body, returns the blood from the parts supplied by the abdominal aorta. It commences at the entrance of the pelvic cavity, runs forward under the bodies of the vertebrae, and empties its blood into the *right atrium* along with that from the anterior vena cava.

78. The contraction of the heart sends the blood out in waves and causes a temporary increased distention of the walls of the arteries. These waves pass from the heart toward the extremities and can be felt where the arteries are near the surface. The waves, or beats, are called the *pulse* and correspond to the contractions of the heart. The normal pulse rate is from 36 to 40 beats a minute.

The Lymphatic System.

79. The lymphatic system consists of a series of vessels, a number of glands through which the vessels pass, and certain fluids known as *lymph* and *chyle*.

80. The lymph vessels are thin, delicate tubes, similar to veins, which gather the lymph from the tissues and convey it to the blood. The lymph from the right fore extremity, the right side of the head, neck, and thorax, is collected by the *right lymphatic vessel*. From all other parts of the body it is collected by the *thoracic duct*; both vessels emptying their lymph into the anterior vena cava just in front of the heart.

81. Lymph glands are small groups of cells through which the lymph vessels pass and in which *white corpuscles* are formed. They also act as filters for the removal of disease germs and other injurious substances.

82. Lymph is a watery fluid by which the tissues are nourished, and by which waste material is gathered from them and eliminated. Lymph is derived from the blood and passes into the tissues by oozing through the thin walls of the capillaries. After bathing and nourishing the tissues it is conveyed by the lymph vessels back to the blood, again. The flow of lymph is brought about by the contraction of the muscles in the vicinity of the vessels.

83. Chyle is a milky fluid formed in the intestines. It contains the nutritive elements of the food and is conveyed by a series of lymph vessels to the blood.

The Nervous System.

84. The nervous system is divided into two minor systems, the *cerebro-spinal*, which is to a considerable extent influenced by the will of the animal, and the *sympathetic*, over which the will has no control.

85. In the *cerebro-spinal* system the central portion is composed of two parts; the *brain*, which occupies the cranial cavity, and the *spinal cord*, which occupies the canal in the vertebrial column. The communicating portion of this system consists of the *cerebro-spinal nerves*, which leave the brain and spinal cord in symmetrical pairs and are distributed to the voluntary muscles and the organs of common sensation and special sense.

86. In the *sympathetic system* the central portion consists of a double chain of *ganglia* (groups of nerve cells) connected by nerves, which extends from the head to the tail below and on each side of the spinal column. The communicating portion of this system is distributed to the involuntary muscles, mucous membranes, internal organs, and blood vessels.

87. A nerve consists of a bundle of tubular fibers, held together by connective tissue. The nerve fibers are simply transmission

lines conveying impressions from the nerve endings to the brain
or cord and conveying impulses from the brain or cord to the muscles

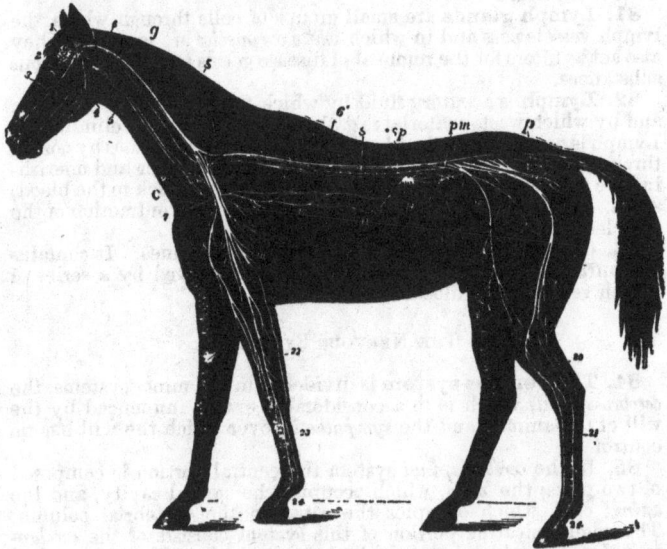

FIG. 17.—Nervous system of the horse. 1, Brain; 2, optic nerve; 3, maxillary nerve
(fifth), 4, mandibular nerve (fifth), 5, vagus nerve, 6, medulla oblongata. 7, right
brachial plexus; 8, musculo-cutaneous nerve, 9, median nerve; 10, radial nerve;
11, ulnar nerve; 12, vagus nerve, 13, coeliac plexus; 14, semilunar ganglion, 15,
lumbo-sacral plexus; 16, femoral nerve; 17, great sciatic nerve; 18, peroneal nerve;
19, external saphenic nerve; 20, tibial nerve, 21, metatarsal nerve; 22, radial portion
of median nerve, 23, metacarpal nerves, 24, digital branches, s. s., sympathetic chain;
c, inferior cervical plexus; g, gutteral ganglion; Sp., great splanchnic nerve, p. m.,
posterior mesenteric plexus; p, pelvic plexus.—(From Strangeways' Veterinary
Anatomy.)

and various organs. In the cerebro-spinal system these impulses
are considerably influenced by the will of the animal.

The Eye.

88. The eyes are the organs of sight and are situated in the orbital cavities. The eye is spherical in shape and is held in position by muscles which turn it and retract it (draw it back) in the orbital cavity. A *pad* of *fat* below and behind the eye protects it from injury due to blows and causes the *membrana nictitans* to pass over the front of the eye when it is retracted by the muscles.

89. The eye is protected by two movable fleshy curtains, the *upper* and *lower* *eyelids*. These are composed of muscular and fibrous tissue in their central portion and are covered externally with skin. The internal surface of the eyelids, the membrana nictitans and the front part of the eye are covered with a mucous membrane, the *conjunctiva*, which is continuous with the skin at the edges of the eyelids. In the edges of the eyelids are strong hairs which protect the eye from dust and small objects floating in the air.

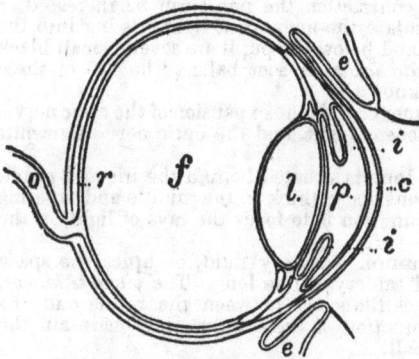

Fig. 18.—Section of the eye. *c*, Cornea, eyelids, *f*, fluid; *i*, iris, *l*, crystalline lens, *o*, optic nerve, *p*, pupil, *r*, retina.

90. The membrana nictitan, or accessory eyelid (haw), is situated between the inner side of the orbital cavity and the eyeball, within the lids. When the eye is retracted it passes over the front part of the eye, removing any foreign objects and moistening the cornea.

91. The eye proper is composed of *three* coats and certain internal structures.

92. The outer covering of the eye is formed by the *sclerotic* coat and the *cornea*. The sclerotic coat is composed of strong white fibrous tissue and forms the protective covering. It covers four-fifths of the eyeball and affords attachment for the muscles of the eye. In front of and continuous with the sclerotic coat is the *cornea*, a transparent tissue which admits the light to the interior of the eye.

93. The choroid, or middle coat, is a vascular membrane of a dark color. At the juncture of the sclerotic coat and the cornea the choroid coat sends down a circular dark colored membrane, the *iris*, in the center of which is the *pupil*, a small opening for the admission of light. By muscular contraction the pupil can be increased or decreased in size to regulate the amount of light passing into the eye. On the iris above and below the pupil are several small black projections called *granula irıdis*, or soot balls. The use of these bodies is not definitely known.

94. The retina, or inner coat, is the expansion of the *optic* nerve. It receives the impressions of sight, and the optic nerve transmits them to the brain.

95. The crystalline lens is situated behind the iris and pupil. It is a circular, transparent body, thick in the middle and tapering toward the edges. Its function is to focus the rays of light on the retina.

96. The aqueous humor, a watery fluid, occupies the space between the cornea and the crystalline lens. The *vitreous humor*, a jellylike fluid, occupies the space between the retina and the crystalline lens. The function of these fluids is to maintain the proper shape of the eyeball.

THE EAR.

97. The ears are the organs of hearing   They are located one on either side of the poll.

98. The ear may be divided into two portions, *external* and *internal*.

99. The external ear is funnel-shaped, formed of cartilage, and covered with skin both inside and outside. There are numerous fine hairs on the inside of the tunnel which prevent the passage of foreign bodies into the internal ear. The lower portion of the funnel communicates with the *internal ear* and is supplied with numerous *sebaceous glands*. There are muscles attached to the lower part of the cartilage by which the ears are moved at will.

100. The internal ear is inclosed in a bony chamber. Here the nerve endings receive the impressions of sound and transmit them to the brain. Separating the internal ear from the external ear is the *tympanum*, or ear drum.

THE SKIN.

101. The skin covers the external surface of the body. It varies in thickness according to the amount of protection the different parts of the body require. The skin is the special organ of touch and is supplied with sensory nerves, particularly at the muzzle and lips. The long hairs (feelers) growing from the muzzle, and in special nerve structures in the dermis.

102. The skin consists of two parts; the outer, called the *epidermis*, or cuticle; and the inner, the *corium*, *dermis*, or true skin.

103. The epidermis is the outer protective covering   The hoof, ergot, and chestnuts are modifications of the epidermis.

104. The dermis lies beneath the inner surface of the epidermis and continually replaces it as it is worm away. It contains the hair follicles, the sebaceous and the sweat glands.

105. Hairs grow from the *hair follicles*, and form the outer protective covering of the body known as the *coat*. The coat is shed twice a year, in the spring and in the fall, and is replaced by a lighter or heavier growth according to the season.

106. The sebaceous glands secrete an oily substance which is formed within them. Where the skin is covered with hair the sebaceous fluid is discharged into the hair follicles   It softens and waterproofs the hair and surrounding skin, keeping them flexible and giving the hair the gloss that is seen in healthy animals. Where no hair is present the glands discharge directly on the surface of the skin, keeping it soft and supple.

107. The sweat glands are groups of cells which excrete sweat. They communicate with the outer surface by simple tubes which pour their excretions on the surface of the skin. *Sweat* consists of water and various salts and waste materials from the blood. It evaporates on the surface of the skin and assists in regulating the temperature of the body.

THE FOOT.

108. The foot is composed of *four parts*: the *bones*; the *elastic structures*; the *corium*; and the *hoof*, the protective organ of the foot.

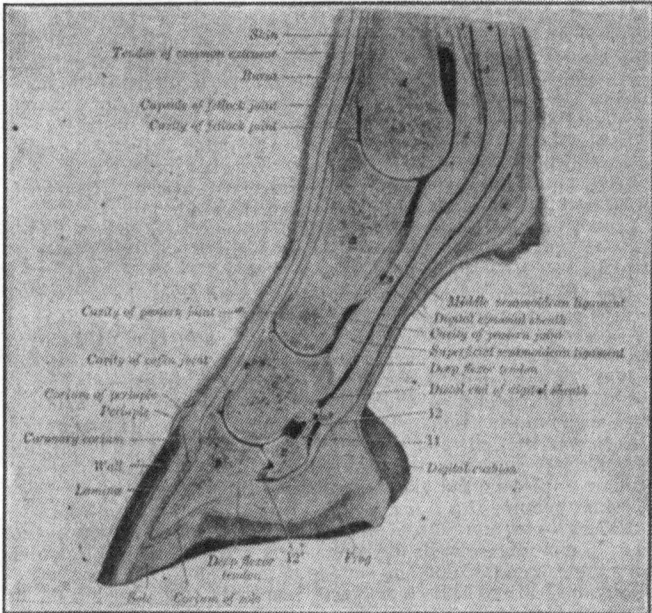

Fig. 19.—Sagittal section of digit and distal part of metacarpus of horse. *A*, Metacarpal bone; *B*, first phalanx, *C*, second phalanx; *D*, third phalanx; *E*, distal sesamoid bone; 1, volar pouch of capsule of fetlock joint; 2, intersesamoidean ligament; 3, 4, proximal end of digital synovial sheath; 5, ring formed by superficial flexor tendon; 6, fibrous tissue underlying ergot; 7, ergot; 8, 9, 9′, branches of digital vessels; 10, distal ligament of distal sesamoid bone; 11, suspensory ligament of distal sesamoid bone; 12, 12′, proximal and distal ends of bursa podotrochlearis. By an oversight the superficial flexor tendon (behind 4) is not marked. (From Sisson's Anatomy of the Domestic Animals; copyright, W. B. Saunders Co.)

BONES OF THE FOOT.

109. The bones of the pastern and foot are the *first phalanx* (long pastern bone), the *second phalanx* (short pastern bone), the *third phalanx* (coffin bone), and the *navicular bone* (distal sesamoid). The first two bones require no description.

110. The third phalanx (coffin bone) is entirely inclosed by the hoof, which it resembles in shape.

The upper or *articular surface* faces upward and backward and articulates with the *second phalanx*. Immediately behind and below this surface is a small area for the articulation of the *navicular* bone.

The *wall surface* (front and sides) slopes downward and forward. It is roughened for the attachment of the *laminar corium* and perforated by numerous small openings for the passage of *blood vessels* and *nerves*. At the top of this surface, in front, is a ridge to which the tendon of the extensor of the foot is attached.

The *under surface* corresponds in shape to the *sole* of the *hoof*. It is smooth except at the back part, which is roughened for the attachment of the tendon of the deep flexor of the foot.

The *wings* (angles) one on either side, project backward and give attachment on their upper borders to the *cartilages* of the *foot*.

111. The navicular bone (distal sesamoid) is shuttle-shaped, and lies behind the junction of the second and third phalanges with which it articulates. The deep flexor tendon of the foot passes over its lower surface.

THE ELASTIC STRUCTURES OF THE FOOT.

112. The cartilages of the third phalanx, also known as the lateral cartilages (fig. 21), are large elastic plates of cartilage, attached one to either wing of the bone. They project backward and upward, their upper borders extending above the hoof, where they may be felt beneath the skin above the coronet at the heels.

113. The digital cushion (plantar cushion) (fig. 19), the principal elastic structure of the foot, is a wedge-shaped pad, situated above the frog, below the deep flexor tendon of the foot, and between the cartilages of the third phalanx. The *apex* or points is directed forward and lies just below the lower end of the deep flexor tendon. The *base* or back part lies under the skin of the heels. The digital cushion acts as a buffer to the foot and prevents jar.

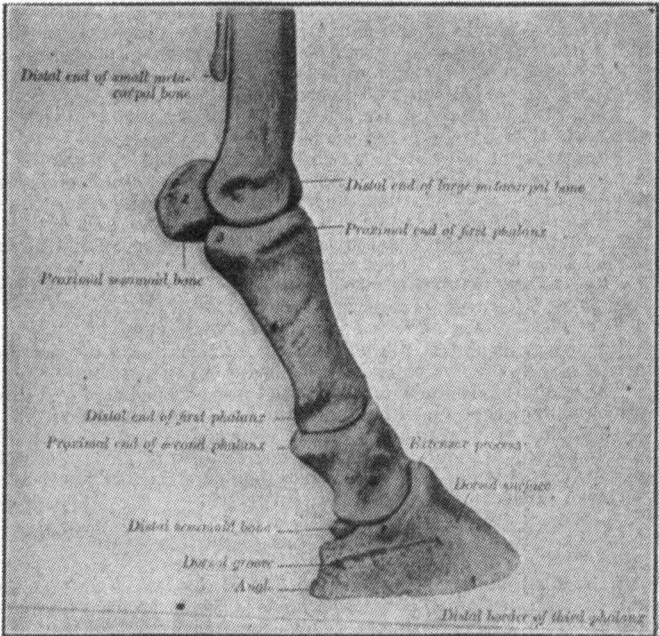

FIG. 20.—Skeleton of digit and distal part of metacarpus of horse, lateral view. 1-7, Eminences and depression for attachment of ligaments. Cartilage of third phalanx is removed. (From Sisson's Anatomy of the Domestic Animals, copyright, W. B. Saunders Co.)

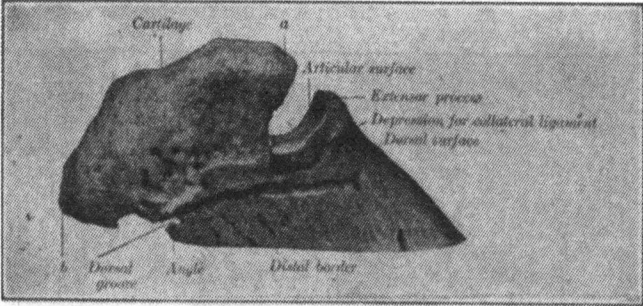

FIG. 21.—Third phalanx of horse, lateral view. *a*, *b*, Anterior and posterior extremities of cartilage. (From Sisson's Anatomy of the Domestic Animals; copyright, W. B. Saunders Co.)

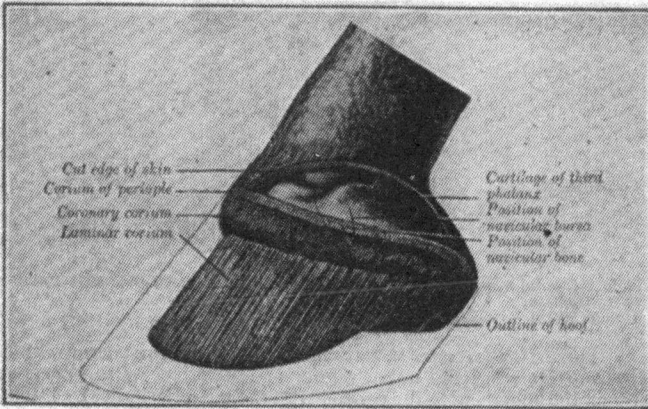

FIG. 22.—Lateral view of foot of horse after removal of hoof and part of skin. (After Schmaltz, Atlas d. Anat. d. Pferdes.) Dotted lines in front of navicular bone indicate position of coffin joint. (From Sisson's Anatomy of the Domestic Animals; copyright, W. B. Saunders Co.)

THE CORIUM.

114. The corium of the hoof is the highly vascular part of the corium or dermis of the skin which completely covers the coffin bone, the digital cushion, and a large surface of the cartilages of the foot. It furnishes nutrition to the hoof, and is divided into five parts which nourish corresponding parts of the hoof

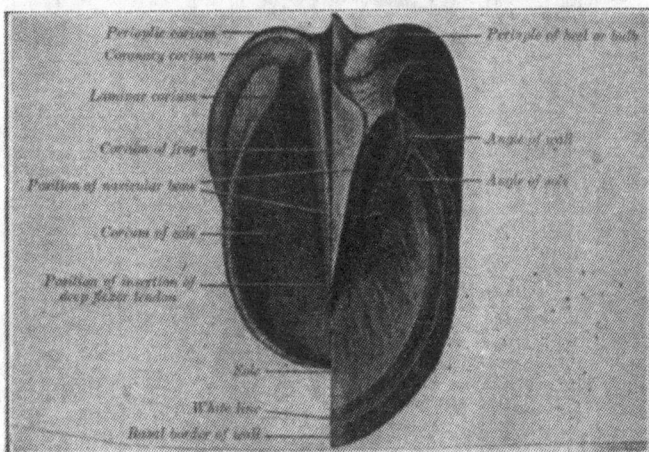

Fig. 23.—Ground surface of foot of horse after removal of half of hoof to show corium. (After Schmaltz, Atlas d. Anat. d. Pferdes.) (From Sisson's Anatomy of the Domestic Animals; copyright, W. B. Saunders Co)

(a) The *perioplic corium* or *ring* (figs. 22, 23) is a narrow band which lies in a groove at the upper border of the wall. At the heels it widens and blends with the corium of the frog. It supplies nutrition to the periople.

(b) The *coronary corium* or *ring* (figs. 22, 23) is a thick band which occupies the coronary groove on the inside of the upper border of the wall. It furnishes nutrition to the bulk of the wall.

(c) The *laminar corium* (sensitive laminae) (fig. 22) is attached to the wall surface of the third phalanx and to the lower part of its cartilages. It bears numerous delicate folds or laminae which

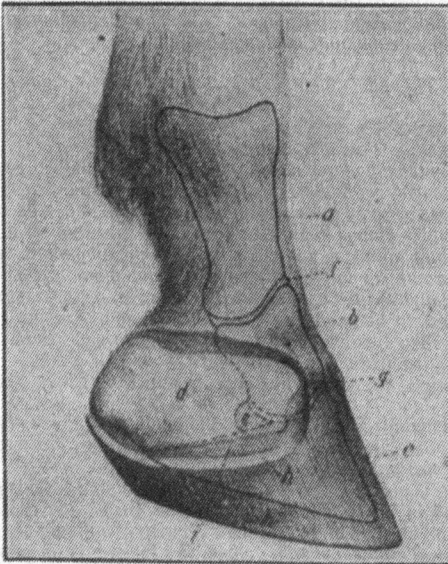

FIG. 24.—Digit of horse, showing surface relations of bones and joints. The cartilage is largely exposed. *a*, First phalanx; *b*, second phalanx, *c*, third phalanx; *d*, cartilage; *e*, distal sesamoid or navicular bone; *f*, pastern joint; *g*, coffin joint; *h'*, cut edge of wall of hoof (*h*); *i*, laminar corium. (After Ellenberger in Leisering's Atlas.) (From Sisson's Anatomy of the Domestic Animals; copyright, W. B. Saunders Co.)

interleave with the horny laminae of the wall and bars. They (the laminae of the corium) supply nourishment to the horny laminae and to the horn of the white line. By their intimate union with the laminae of the wall they support the weight of the body within the hoof.

(*d*) The *corium* of the *sole* (sensitive sole) (figs. 19, 23) corresponds to the horny sole, to which is supplies nutrition.

(*e*) The *corium* of the *frog* (sensitive frog) (fig. 23) is molded on the upper surface of the frog and is attached to the under surface of the digital cushion. It nourishes the frog.

THE HOOF.

115. The hoof is the horny covering of the foot. It is divided into three parts, the *wall*, *sole*, and *frog*.

(*a*) The *wall* is that part of the hoof which is visible when the foot is placed on the ground. It covers the front and sides of the foot, and is bent abruptly inward and forward at the heels to form the *bars*. The latter appear on the bottom of the foot as horny ridges which extend forward and inward toward the point of the frog. The bars secure a solid bearing for the back part of the foot; they give additional strength to the hoof, and, being a part of the wall, are intended to bear weight. For convenience in study the wall may be divided into three parts, the *toe*, *quarters*, and *heels*.

The *toe* is the front part of the wall.

The *quarters*, one on either side, extend backward from the toe to the heels.

The *heels* are the hindermost part of the foot. They are located at the point where the wall bends inward to become the bars.

The *external surface* is smooth, and its upper portion is covered with a thin layer of soft horn called the *periople*. Extending from the periople to the bottom of the foot is a thin layer of horny scales which gives the surface of the wall its smooth, glossy appearance.

The *internal surface* is concave from side to side, and presents about 600 thin, white, parallel plates of horn called *laminae*, which extend from the coronary groove to the bottom of the wall. These horny laminae dovetail with the corresponding laminae of the corium and bind the wall of the hoof to the third phalanx and the greater part of its cartilages.

The *upper* or *coronary border* is thin, and its outer surface is covered by the periople. The inner side of this border is hollowed out to form the *coronary groove*, which extends all the way round the top of the wall and contains the thick *coronary corium*.

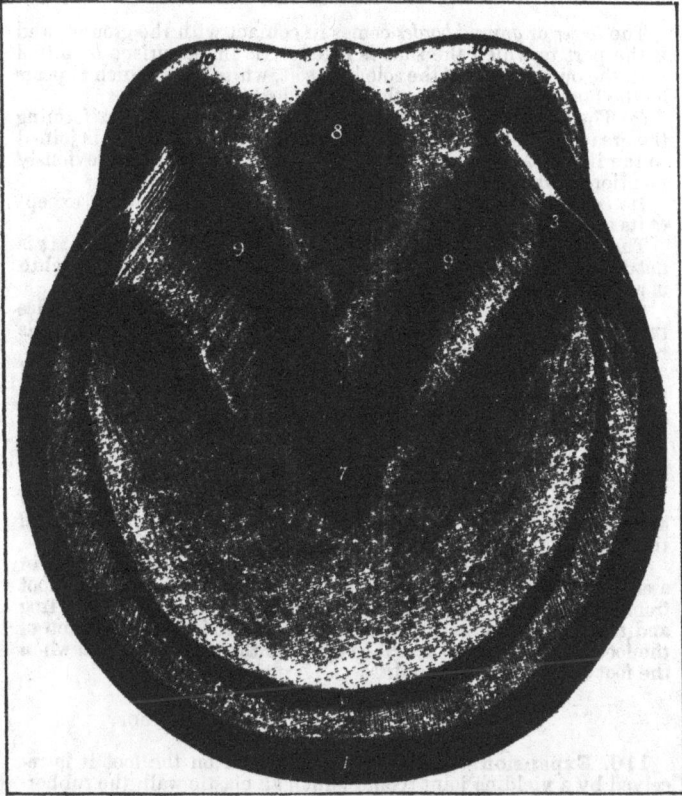

FIG. 25.—Right fore hoof of horse, ground surface. *1,* Basal or ground border of wall; *2,* laminae of wall; *3,* angle of wall, *4,* bar; *5,* sole, *5',* angle of sole; *6,* white line (junction of wall and sole); *7,* apex of frog, *8,* central sulcus of frog, *9, 9,* collateral sulci between frog and bars; *10, 10,* bulbs of hoof. (From Sisson's Anatomy of the Domestic Animals; copyright, W. B. Saunders Co.)

The *lower* or *ground border* comes in contact with the ground, and is the part to which the shoe is fitted. Its inner surface is united with the outer border of the sole by a soft, white horn, which appears on the bottom of the foot as the so-called *white line*.

(*b*) The *sole* is a thick, half-moon-shaped plate of horn forming the greater part of the bottom of the foot. *Its outer border* is joined to the inner part of the lower border of the wall by the previously mentioned white line.

Its *inner border* is V-shaped, and is attached to the *bars*, except at its narrow part, where it joins the point of the frog.

The use of the sole is to protect the sensitive parts above. It is not intended to bear weight, except on a margin about one-eighth of an inch wide inside of the white line.

(*c*) The *frog* is a wedge-shaped mass of soft horn which occupies the V-shaped space bounded by the bars and sole, and extends below these on the bottom of the foot.

On the *lower* or *ground surface* are two prominent ridges, separated behind by a cavity called the *cleft*, and joined in front to form the *apex* or point of the frog.

The *base* or *posterior extremity* is depressed in the center and bulged at the sides, where it unites with the wall at the heels, forming two round prominences called the *bulbs* of the *hoof*.

The *upper surface* of the frog is the exact reverse of the lower and shows a middle ridge, the *spine* or *frog-stay*. Between the sides of the frog and the bars are two cavities called the *commissures*.

The frog protects the sensitive structures above, acts as a pad in assisting the digital cushion in breaking jar, and prevents the foot from slipping. The frog-stay forms a firm union between the frog and the frog corium above. It may also assist in the expansion of the foot by being forced like a wedge into the digital cushion when the foot comes to the ground.

EXPANSION AND CONTRACTION OF THE HOOF.

116. Expansion.—When weight is placed on the foot it is received by a yielding joint (coffin joint), an elastic wall, the rubber-like frog, the digital cushion, and the more or less yielding sole. The digital cushion and the frog are compressed between the ground below and the structures above, which causes them to spread out sidewise, carrying with them the cartilages and bars and the wall at the quarters. This is called *expansion*, and amounts to about one-twenty-fifth of an inch total increase in width of the foot at the heel.

117. Contraction.—When weight is removed from the foot, the digital cushion and frog return to their normal shape, and the cartilages and quarters move inward to where they were before expansion occurred. This is called *contraction*.

118. The benefits derived from these movements are many; they diminish jar or shock to the foot and leg, and prevent the evil results of concussion; they increase the elasticity of the entire limb, and assist in the circulation of the blood in the foot.

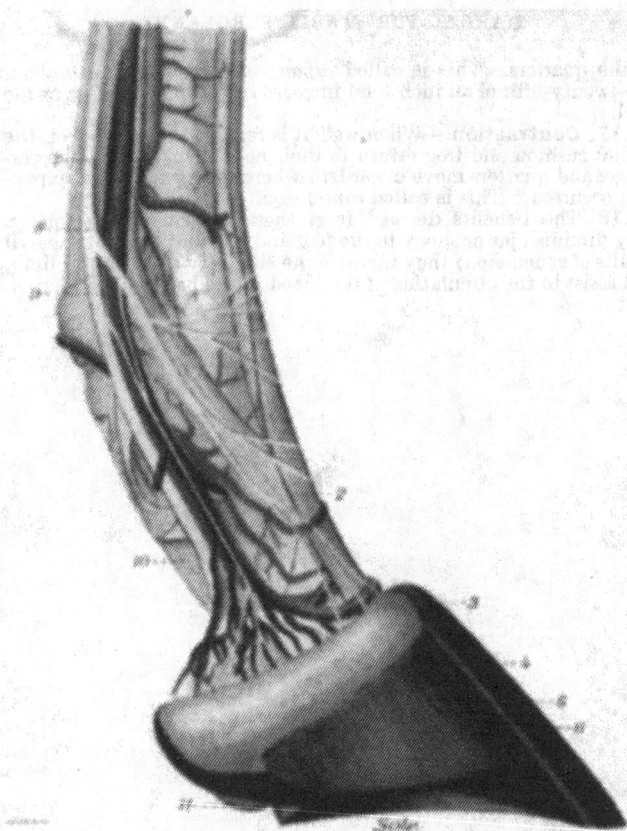

FIG. 26.—FOOT OF THE HORSE.

1, Metacarpal bone ; *2*, extensor tendon ; *3*, coronary corium ; *4*, laminar corium ; *5*, wall ; *6*, laminae ; *7*, volar nerve ; *8*, metacarpal vein ; *9*, digital artery ; *10*, superficial flexor tendon ; *11*, frog. (From "Diseases of the Horse," U. S. Department of Agriculture.

CHAPTER II.

NAMES AND CONFORMATION OF EXTERNAL REGIONS—APPEARANCES OF HEALTH.

NAMES AND CONFORMATION OF EXTERNAL REGIONS.

119. The external regions and structures of the body should present the following appearances:

HEAD AND NECK

Head.—Clear cut, lean, straight, and of proportionate size.

Forehead.—Broad, full, and flat.

Face.—Straight. When convex (bulging) the horse is said to have a *Roman nose.* A concave (hollow) face is called a *dish face.*

Lower jaw.—Wide and strong, with plenty of space between its branches for the larynx.

Muzzle.—The muzzle includes the nostrils and the lips.

Lips.—Small, thin, and firm.

Nostrils.—Large and free from coarse hairs in their entrances.

Eyes.—Large, clear, bright, prominent, and free from cloudiness and spots; lids thin, well open, and evenly curved.

Ears—Medium size, pointed, fine, set moderately close, and carried erect.

Poll.—Smooth and free from enlargements and scars.

Throat and parotid region.—Clean and free from swollen or enlarged glands.

Neck.—Of moderate length, well muscled, clean, well arched, nicely set on, and not too narrow just in rear of the throat; windpipe large and prominent; a neck with a concave upper border is known as an *ewe neck.*

Mane.—Fine and silky.

Jugular channel.—Free from enlargements, smooth, and clean.

120. Forehand.

Withers.—Extending well back, muscular, neither too high nor too low, and free from scars.

Shoulders.—For cavalry horses, long, sloping, and well muscled. For artillery and draft horses, they should be more nearly upright and their front line clearly marked with a smooth, even surface and free from excessive muscular development at a point marked "A," figure 27, which prevents a close fit of the collar.

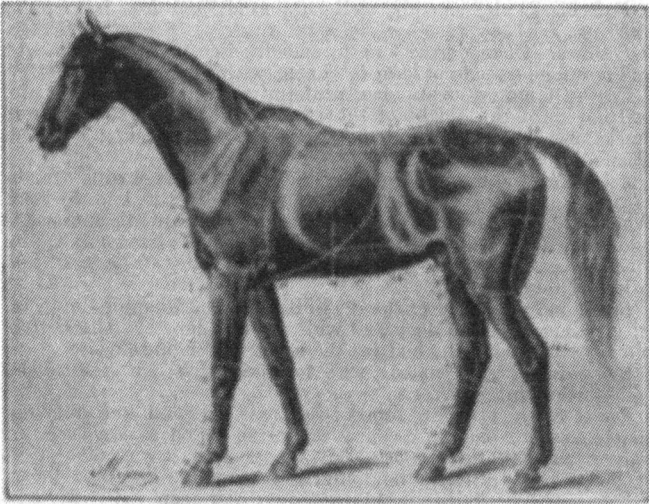

FIG. 27.—External regions of the horse. 1, Lips; 2, muzzle; 3, face; 4, forehead; 5, eyebrows; 6, forelock; 7, ears; 8, lower jaw; 9, cheek; 10, nostril; 11, poll; 11a, throat; 12, parotid; 13, neck; 13a, mane; 14, jugular channel; 15, breast (front of chest); 16, withers; 17, back; 18, ribs, or barrel; 19, girth; 20, loins; 21, croup; 22, tail; 23, dock; 24, flank; 25, belly; 26, sheath; 27, testicles; 28, point of shoulder; 28a, shoulder; 28b, arm; 29, elbow; 30, forearm; 31, chestnut; 32, knee; 33, cannon; 34, fetlock joint; 35, pastern; 36, coronet; 37, foot; 38, fetlock; 39, haunch (point of hip); 40, thigh; 41, stifle; 42, buttock; 43, gaskin; 44, hock; 44a, point of hock; 45, chestnut; 46, cannon; 47, fetlock joint; 48, fetlock; 49, pastern; 50, coronet. 51, foot.

Arms.—Short, muscular, and set well forward.
Elbows.—Large and long and clear of the chest.
Forearms.—Long, broad, and well muscled.

Knees.—Straight, broad, deep, and free from puffiness, scars and swellings. A knee bent backwards is called a *calf knee.* The opposite condition is known as *knee-sprung* or *over in the knees.*

Cannons.—Short, broad, flat, and of uniform size. Tendons smooth, and well set back. If smaller below the knee than elsewhere, the leg is said to be *tied in* below the knee.

Fetlocks.—Wide, smooth, well supported, and free from puffy swellings.

Pasterns.—Of moderate length, smooth, free from enlargements, and forming an angle of form 45° to 50° with the ground.

Feet.—Of proportionate size, uniform, and circular, heels wide, and one-third the height of the toe; walls smooth and free from cracks, fissures, and rings; bars strong, sole concave, frog large and elastic, horn dense and tough.

Legs.—Viewed from the front, vertical, with toes pointing straight to the front. Viewed from the side, slightly inclined to the rear. When the toe points obliquely forward and inward, the animal is said to be *pigeon-toed.* The opposite condition is known as *toe out* or *splay footed.*

121. Body.

Breast and chest.—Of moderate width and considerable depth for cavalry horses. Both deep and wide for draft horses. The girth is the measure around the body at the chest. It should be large.

Ribs.—Long, well arched, close together. Last rib close to the point of the hip.

Back.—Short, straight, broad, well muscled, and free from enlargements and scars. A concave back is called a *sway back.* A convex back is called a *roach back.*

Loins.—Broad, short, strong, and well muscled.

Flanks.—Close, full (not hollowed out), and deep.

Underline of the chest and belly.—Long and well let down. When this line passes obliquely backward and upward, the horse is said to be *herring gutted.*

122. Hindquarters.

Croup.—Long, rounded, and sloping slightly downward. When it droops and becomes narrow below the tail the horse is said to be *goose rumped.*

Haunch (*point of hip*).—Not too prominent, yet not drooped or sunken.

Dock.—Large and muscular.

Tail.—Set fairly high, and carried well away from the body. Hairs fine and silky.

Thighs and buttocks.—Long and muscular, muscles extending well down into the gaskin. When the muscles of the inner side of the thighs are but little developed, the horse is said to be *split up behind*.

Stifles.—Large, broad, well muscled, and free from puffiness.

Gaskins.—Long, broad, and muscular.

Hocks.—Large, wide, deep from front to rear, smooth, well supported, and free from puffy swellings and bony enlargements; point prominent, clean, and standing well away from the joint. The hocks should stand well apart, but not enough to give the horse the appearance of being *bow-legged*. When the hocks stand close together and the hind feet well apart, with the toes turned out, the horse is said to be *cow hocked*. The term *sickle hock* is applied to hocks that appear overly bent when viewed from the side.

Cannons.—Short, wide, and flat; tendons smooth and well defined, and the line from the point of the hock to the fetlock straight, and nearly perpendicular.

Fetlocks —Large, wide, well supported, and free from puffy swellings. When the fetlock is inclined too far forward, the condition is called *cocked ankle*.

Pasterns.—Of moderate length, large, free from enlargements, and inclined at an angle of from 50° to 55° with the ground.

Feet.—Same as fore feet, except that the shape is oval, the sole more concave, and the wall more nearly vertical.

Appearances of Health.

123. Manner of standing.—Fore feet square and firm on the ground; one hind foot may or may not be resting on the toe. A fore leg is never rested unless injured, diseased, or greatly fatigued. In the latter condition the feet are alternately lifted and replaced in position by a slow and regular stamping movement. The head is held erect, the eyes are wide open and there is a lively play of the ears.

124. Skin.—Loose, supple, and easily moved about over the structures beneath.

125. Coat.—Smooth, sleek, and glossy. In cold weather, unless blankets are used, the hair stands upright, the coat becomes heavy and coarse and loses its gloss.

126. Pulse.—Strong, full, regular, and beating from 36 to 40 times a minute. The number of beats is increased by exercise, excitement, and disease.

The pulse is taken by placing the fore or middle finger transversely (crosswise) on the submaxillary artery at the margin of the lower jaw, and counting the pulsations for half a minute and then multiplying the result by two.

127. Respiration.—Free, soft, and noiseless. Number of respirations per minute.

At rest	10–12
Walking 200 yards	28
Trotting 5 minutes	52
Galloping 5 minutes	52

After exercise the breathing should subside quickly to normal. The ratio of respiration to the beat of the heart is about one respiration to four heartbeats.

The respirations are counted by watching the rise and fall of the flank, the movements of the nostrils, or, on a cold day, the steamy expiration of the breath.

128. Temperature.—Varies from 99° to 100° F. It is increased by exercise, excitement, and disease. Age has a slight influence, the temperature being higher in young animals and lower in old ones. In the Tropics it may average as high as 100.5° F.

The temperature is taken with a clinical thermometer in the rectum. The thermometer is moistened or oiled, the mercury is shaken down to 96 or below, and the bulb of the thermometer is inserted into the anus, and allowed to remain three minutes, when it is withdrawn and the temperature noted.

129. Defecation—Occurs from 10 to 12 times in 24 hours, the droppings being fairly well formed, free from offensive odor, and varying in color from yellow to green, according to the nature of the food. The amount of feces passed in 24 hours varies from 36 to 40 pounds, depending upon the size of the animal and the amount of food given.

130. Urination.—Urine is passed several times daily, in quantities of a quart or more. It is a thick yellowish fluid, and the quantity passed in 24 hours varies from 3 to 6 quarts. During the act of urination horses straddle, grunt, and assume a very awkward position, which must not be mistaken for pain.

CHAPTER III.

STABLE HYGIENE—CARE OF THE SICK AND INJURED.

Stable Hygiene.

131. Ventilation.—The object of ventilation is to supply pure air to the lungs, to dilute and remove the products of respiration, and the ordor and gases arising from the fluid and solid excrements which have been evacuated by the occupants of the building.

132. Composition of air.—Pure air consists of:

	Parts.
Oxygen	2,096
Nitrogen	7,900
Carbonic acid	4
Total	10,000

It also contains a small quantity of watery vapor.

Oxygen is the chief useful part of the air for purifying the blood. *Nitrogen* dilutes the oxygen and renders it respirable. The amount of *carbonic acid* is very small, but if it rises beyond 6 parts in 10,000 the air is impure and unfit to breathe.

Air is rendered *impure* by the respiration of men and animals, its carbonic acid and watery vapor are increased, its oxygen diminished, and a proportion of organic matter added to it. So long as respiration is occurring in the open air these impurities are gotten rid of as fast as they are formed, but in the air of buildings it is different, for here they accumulate unless means are at hand for getting rid of them. The employment of such means is known as ventilation.

133. Testing the ventilation.—The proper time to test the ventilation is in the morning before the doors are opened. If on entering the stable a sense of stuffiness is detected, the ventilation is defective, and more air must be supplied.

134. Draft and chill.—A draft is a current of air passing through a confined space, such as a window or door, at such a rate as to produce a feeling of cold when it strikes the skin. The effect of such a draft on a warm skin is to drive the blood into the internal organs and produce chill and shivering. Tying animals in a draft must therefore be carefully avoided.

135. Windows and roof ventilators.—In calm weather the windows and ventilators should always be kept open. During storms they should be closed on the windward side only. When the storm ceases they should all be opened again. In warm weather the doors should also be kept open.

136. Temperature of stable air.—Horses suffer very little from cold; they stand changes of temperature remarkably well, and chills from standing in a draft when heated and tired are the only changes of temperature which are likely to produce sickness. Stables are therefore not intended to keep animals warm, but to protect them from draft and storm.

Hot stables produce a fine glossy coat, cause the animals to put on fat, but also lower their vitality and increase their susceptibility to disease. Cold stables produce a rough heavy coat, there is not much tendency to put on fat, and the animals require more to eat, owing to the increased demand on the heat-producing function. They are healthier, however, and better able to stand exposure and hardships, such as animals of the military service may at any time be called upon to do.

When new horses are put for the first time in the stable, or when older horses return from maneuvers or duty in the field, the greatest care should be taken with regard to ventilation. Every door and every window should be left open or for a certainty they will contract a catarrh.

137. Care of stalls and floors.—As soon as the horses are through feeding in the morning they should be removed from the stable and the stalls thoroughly cleaned. At the same time the doors and windows should be opened to thoroughly air and dry out the building.

Mangers and feed boxes must be kept clean. Hay and grain that have been left in them should be removed and the boxes washed at least once a week, and always after bran mashes have been fed.

The bedding is carefully shaken out and sorted, and all parts which can be used again are put to one side.

Manure and waste bedding must be taken to the manure heap daily.

138. Cement, brick, and stone floors, during warm weather and in the Tropics, are best cleaned by scrubbing with water, using the hose and stable brooms where available, the floors being allowed to dry before putting down the bedding. In cold weather this is not practicable, and the cleaning should be done by scraping with a hoe or shovel and sweeping with a stable broom.

If the floors become slippery from ice, sand or sifted ashes should be put on them before the bedding is put down; this to prevent injury to the horses from slipping.

Should the floors wear smooth and become slippery, the surface should be roughened by chipping with a stone or cold chisel and mallet. The chisel can be made by the troop blacksmith.

When for any purpose the horses are tied in during the day, the stalls should be cleaned again as soon as the horses are turned out.

139. Dirt floors.—Dirt floors require continual work to keep them in good condition. As soon as wet spots or depressions form they should be dug out and filled with fresh clay well wet and tamped in. The front of the stall floor should be 2 inches higher than the floor at the rear.

140. Bedding.—The monthly allowance of bedding is 100 pounds of straw or hay for each horse, or 3⅓ pounds daily. To give animals a good bed, this must be used as economically as possible.

During pleasant weather all parts of the bedding which can be used again are taken out and spread on the bedding racks to dry. In the evening it is returned to the stalls and enough fresh straw or bedding added to make a comfortable bed. Habitually the bedding should be put down just before the horses are tied in for the night. Putting it down in the morning prevents the stalls drying out and allows the stable police to conceal the fact that they have neglected to clean the stables properly.

141. Care of the corral.—The corral should be cleaned twice a day, once at morning stables and again in the evening after the horses have been tied in for the night.

Thorough drainage should be provided, and all depressions kept filled, so that after rains no pools of standing water may remain.

The picket line should be drawn tight and raised high enough so that the horses can not rub themselves on it. Seven feet from the ground is about the proper height. The fastenings at the end of the line should be outside the corral.

The floor of the picket line should be raised and trenches to carry off the rain should be provided so that the ground on which the horses stand may be kept dry.

142. Water troughs.—Water troughs should be emptied and thoroughly cleaned each morning. Under no circumstances should strange animals be permitted to drink at the water trough or be fed in the stable, as one animal with a contagious disease may infect all the animals of the organization.

143. Grooming.—Grooming is essential to the health and appearance of the domesticated horse. Its objects are cleanliness, prevention of disease, particularly of the skin, and the improvement of the animal's general condition. While many diseases are not the direct result of dirt, it is nevertheless true that they are most frequently found where dirty conditions prevail.

Horses should be thoroughly groomed at least once a day, and this should be immediately after exercise or work. They should also be brushed off before going to drill or exercise.

The *idle horse* should be groomed the same as the rest

Mud should be wisped off with hay or straw, or it should be allowed to dry, then removed with a brush.

144. Wet horses.—Wet horses should be dried before being groomed or left tied-up to the line or in the stable. If wet from rain or by washing, wisping with loose straw and lively rubbing with grooming rags or pieces of gunny sacking is a good method of making them dry and warm.

145. Sweating horses.—Sweating horses should be blanketed and walked about until cool, then rubbed and wisped until dry. Returning horses from work wet with sweat may be avoided by allowing them to walk the last half mile or so of the return journey.

146. Hand rubbing.—Hand rubbing is most soothing and restful to tired muscles and limbs. It also removes the loose hair and produces a smooth glossy coat.

To remove hair and stimulate the skin, the hands are slapped down briskly on the coat one after the other, the weight of the body is thrown against them, while both are moved over the skin with firm pressure.

The legs should be rubbed briskly with the fingers and palms in the direction of the hair. After rubbing, the legs should be carefully bandaged, taking care that the bandages are not too tight.

147. Washing horses.—As a general practice this should not be allowed except in warm climates, and then only when the temperature of the air and the water used is approximately the same as that of the body. In cold and changeable climates washing may cause chilling and lead to sickness, usually respiratory diseases and chapping of the skin.

When horses are washed, great care must be taken that they are thoroughly dried by wisping and rubbing and that they are not exposed to drafts before being dried. Washing mud off the legs and belly frequently results in such diseases as scratches, grease heel, and mud fever. These conditions are not caused by the mud, but are the result of improperly drying the legs after washing. When mud can not be wisped off with hay or straw it should be allowed to dry, then removed with a brush. If for any reason the legs must be washed they should be dried and bandaged loosely with flannel bandages. When the bandages are removed the legs should be hand rubbed thoroughly.

Soap should not be used on the legs, as this removes the natural greasiness of the coat and irritates the skin.

148. Clipping.—Clipping in the spring is especially advisable, and in individual cases and under certain circumstances it may become a necessity; but no horse should be clipped without authority from the organization commander. In winter a clipped horse should be provided with a blanket at all times when not working. Under no circumstances should a horse be blanketed while at work.

Horses taken from cold regions to the Tropics still develop their winter coats. Under such conditions clipping is a necessity.

Should it become necessary to keep horses clipped, they should be clipped at least three times a year; the first time in October or November, again in January, and a third time in March or April or just before the spring shedding of the coat. Better still, the clippers should be run over the coat every time it appears at all long.

In clipping the legs, care should be taken not to cut the short hairs at the back of the pasterns or in the hollows of the heels. These hairs when clipped irritate the skin and may cause scratches.

149. Blanketing.—Horses stand changes of temperature and inclement weather remarkably well. Blankets therefore are not absolutely essential to the animal's health.

In garrison and camp, except in extremely cold climates, the use of blankets should be limited to animals that have been clipped, and to those that have become chilled, wet, or heated. They should be worn in the stable or camp only, and should never be permitted while horses are at exercise or work.

All blankets should be shaken daily and aired.

150. Care of the feet.—The healthy foot requires only to be kept clean. In cold climates the feet need be cleaned but once a day; but in hot, damp climates, where there is a great amount of decomposing matter in the soil, they should be well cleaned out both morning and evening. The evening cleaning should be done after the horses are tied in for the night.

The cleaning is done with the hoof-hook, the point of which should be blunted so as not to tear away the horn of the commissures and cleft of the frog.

151. Cleaning the sheath.—The sheath should be cleaned occasionally by washing. Some horses require it more often than others, and especially is it required during hot and dusty weather. In the Tropics and during certain seasons of the year, the presence of screw-worms and maggots from the attacks of flies renders close attention to this detail very necessary. In some horses a thick cheesy-like substance accumulates at the end of the penis on either side of the urethra forming the so-called bean, which may interfere with urination.

The bean should be carefully removed and the penis and inside of the sheath well cleaned with warm water and castile soap. When the parts are thoroughly cleaned, rinse with a warm creolin solution (1-100) and dry. In cold weather drying must be done with great care in order to prevent chilling. To avoid injuring the sheath and penis, the finger nails of the man doing the washing must be cut short and made smooth.

152. Salting.—A lump of salt should be kept in each feed box. If salt is kept in the corral, it should be in a waterproof box protected from rain, for if exposed to moisture it will melt and run on the ground. The ground becoming salty around the box, the horses acquire the habit of licking it and eating the dirt.

Loose salt only should be given in the field.

The daily allowance of salt for each public animal is 0.8 ounce.

153. Water.—A horse requires from 5 to 15 gallons of water daily, depending upon the temperature and the amount of work he is doing. On board ship 10 gallons daily should be provided.

Water should be *fresh, pure,* and *clear,* and *free* from *taste, color,* and *smell.*

154. Watering.—Horses should be watered before feeding, or, if this is impossible, not until two hours after feeding. They may be watered while at work, but, if hot, they should be kept moving until cooled off.

In temperate climates, horses should be watered three times a day, morning, noon, and evening.

In the Tropics and during warm weather, horses, except when they are heated, should have free access to water at all times.

In winter, horses that are tired or heated should be given water that has been slightly warmed. In warm weather and in the Tropics, they may at all times be permitted to drink freely of water that is of the same temperature as that of the air.

In taking horses to water, they should go at a walk. There should be no crowding or hurrying, and each animal should be given plenty of time to drink his fill.

In camp, where water is obtained from a river or a stream, horses must be watered above the place designated for bathing and for washing clothing.

In watering from streams whose bottoms are of mud or fine sand, causing the water to become roily, buckets or improvised troughs should be used.

155. Feeding.—Forage is any food suitable for horses and can be divided into two general classes, hay and grain. The ration must be sufficiently bulky to keep the stomach and intestines partially filled at all times, as the process of digestion is best carried out in this state. Without sufficient bulk, conditions can not be maintained, no matter how nourishing the food.

The capacity of the horse's stomach is small in comparison to his size. He therefore requires to be fed frequently.

156. Feeding tired horses.—Exhausting work has a temporary weakening effect on the digestion, and tired horses should be allowed to recover from its effect before they are given a heavy feed of grain. Give such animals plenty of tepid water, a few pounds of hay, and good care until the system has recovered from exhaustion.

Animals that have been kept from food for a long time should first be watered and given a small feed of hay to partially fill the stomach before feeding grain.

157. Feeding hay.—It is best not to give any hay at the feed immediately preceding the time at which animals are to be required for work, especially work at the fast gaits. When the work is done mostly in the morning, 3 to 4 pounds of hay may be fed to advantage with the noon feed of grain, the remainder of the hay ration being given with the evening feed.

158. Feeding grain.—Grain should be fed three times daily, giving the largest feed at night. Should it become necessary to change the grain ration, as from oats to corn, the allowance of grain should be cut down to one-half, and the amount gradually increased until the animals become accustomed to it. When two different grains, such as corn and oats, are issued, they should be fed separately, feeding the corn at night as it takes longer to thoroughly masticate and digest it. If corn and oats are fed together, the corn being the harder will not be properly masticated, and a portion of its nutriment will be lost. To get the best results, horses should be fed at regular hours, and it is absolutely necessary that the food be pure, clean, and sound.

159. Time required for eating.—It takes a horse from 5 to 10 minutes to eat 1 pound of grain, and from 15 to 20 minutes to eat 1 pound of hay.

160. The forage ration.—The forage ration for a horse is 14 pounds of hay and 12 pounds of oats, corn, or barley; for a field artillery horse of the heavy draft type weighing 1,300 pounds or over, 17 pounds of hay and 14 pounds of oats, corn, or barley; for a mule, 14 pounds of hay and 9 pounds of oats, corn, or barley. To each animal 3 pounds of bran may be issued in lieu of that quantity of grain.

161. Hay.—Hay is any good grass cut at the proper time and well cured.

162. Characteristics of good hay.—Good hay should be moderately fine, somewhat hard to the touch, sound, sweet smelling, well cured, and free from weeds. The color should be a bright natural green, and should give an idea of newness. The flowering heads of the grasses ought to be present and should not shell out when rubbed. When chewed, it should have a mild, pleasant taste.

163. Defects in hay.—Hay may be badly cured, overripe, mow burned, caked in the bale, dusty, musty, or moldy. All such hay is unfit to use and should be put aside and reported to the organization commander.

164. Badly saved hay.—Badly saved hay is such as results from getting wet while being cured. If not dusty or moldy, it may be fed, but it does not have the full nutritive value.

165. Overripe hay.—Overripe hay is yellow, dry, and hard, with the leaves broken off and the heads shelled out. Such hay is of no more value than straw.

166. Mow-burned hay.—Mow-burned hay is the result of overheating in the stack, due to being stored away while damp. Such hay varies in color from light brown to dark, or almost black. The stalk is dry and brittle with a bitter, pungent odor and taste. Such hay should not be used as it may produce digestive derangements and kidney diseases.

167. Hay caked in the bale.—Baled hay that externally has a good appearance but does not spring apart when the wires are taken off has been baled wet, and presents the same appearance as mow-burned hay. Such hay is unfit for use.

168. Dusty hay.—Dusty hay, due to gradual dry decay from long exposure to the sun or attacks of insects, produces dry coughs and digestive derangements and should not be used.

169. Musty and moldy hay.—Musty or moldy hay is readily recognized by the presence of the white mold on the leaves and stalks; when shaken, it gives off a very irritating dust. This hay is bitter to the taste and its use is dangerous. Where no other hay or roughage is available, it may be used, but it must be opened out and dried, well shaken to get rid of the mold, and wet with salt water—a tablespoonful of salt to a bucket of water. Its effect must be carefully watched and it should be fed only when no other hay can be obtained.

Horses can not be fed on grain alone, so if hay is not obtainable a substitute must be found.

170. Grain hay.—Hay made from oats, wheat, and barley, cut before it is matured is frequently used. Such hay contains a proportion of grain which reduces the bulk of the ration. To allow for this the grain ration should be reduced about 3 pounds and the hay increased the same amount.

171. Straw.—Clean straw of oats, wheat, barley, and rye, and, in the Tropics, rice straw may be fed when hay can not be obtained, but it must be clean, sound, and free from dirt and weeds. Dried corn fodder may also be used as a substitute for hay.

172. Green forage.—When green grass or green corn fodder is fed in lieu of hay, the average proportion allowed is 3 pounds of green food to 1 pound of hay, or 42 pounds of green food daily. Care must be taken that green foods are not piled up and allowed to heat before feeding, for this will cause scouring and colic.

173. Grazing.—Grazing is very beneficial and advantage should be taken of every opportunity to give the horses a bite of grass. In turning horses out for the first time to graze, care must be taken that they do not overeat.

Grazing on wet or frosted alfalfa or clover must not be permitted, as flatulent colic is almost sure to result.

174. Grains.—Grains are not the natural food of the horse, but they are necessary to obtain from horses the maximum amount of energy they are capable of yielding. All grains do not have the same feeding value; oats, corn, and barley have been found to give the best results.

175. Oats.—Oats are the best and most valuable grain for horses. The oat is composed of two parts, the hull or husk and the kernel. The larger the kernel, in proportion to the hull, the better the oat.

The husk is thinner in white oats than in the red and black varieties. The short plump oat is a heavy one, while the longer and more bearded the oat, the lighter it is.

176. Weight of oats.—The legal weight of a bushel of oats is 32 pounds, but northern oats often weigh as much as 45 pounds to the bushel.

177. Feeding oats.—Oats are fed whole, it being only necessary to grind, crush, or steam them for animals with poor teeth.

178. Characteristics of oats.—Oats should be short and plump, of good color, hard to the feel, rattling when poured out on a solid surface, without smell, breaking across when bitten, and having the taste of good oatmeal. They should also be free from dirt, stalks, stems, and seeds of other plants.

179. Defects in oats.—Oats may be clipped, foxy, bleached or sulphured, damp, sprouting, musty, or moldy. All defective grain should be put aside and reported at once.

180. Clipped oats.—Clipped oats are oats from which the beards have been removed by passing them over a revolving screen. This process produces a shorter, plumper looking grain, which packs better and weighs more to the bushel. The cut ends may be seen, and if the hand is put deep into the sack the clipped beards may be found adhering to it on removal. If such oats are clean and sound, the process does not detract from their value as a food.

181. Foxy oats.—When oats are stored before they are sufficiently dried, they become heated, their color is changed to a deep yellow or brown, both the husk and the kernel, and they acquire a peculiar bitter odor and taste. Such oats are termed *foxy*. They are unfit for food.

182. Bleached or sulphured oats.—Foxy oats are sometimes bleached with the fumes of sulphur to destroy their color and smell, but the process does not remove the stain or bitter taste from the kernel. To detect this fraud, rub a small quantity of the suspected oats between the palms of the hands until they become warm, or heat over a fire; when warmed they give off the characteristic odor of sulphur. Such oats are not fit to use.

183. Damp oats.—When oats have been wet and sufficient time has not elapsed to allow of their heating and spoiling, they may be fed, even though soft.

184. Sprouting oats.—Such oats are unfit for food.

185. Musty oats.—Mustiness is a condition resulting from dampness. Musty oats are easily recognized by their softened,

discolored kernel and hull, and their bitter and musty taste and
smell. They are unfit for food, and are sometimes poisonous,
producing diseases of the digestive organs and kidneys.

186. Moldy oats.—Moldy oats are in a state of positive decay,
and are absolutely unfit for food. They are recognized by their
softened, rotten condition, and by the presence of the mold on
the hull.

187. Corn.—Corn is a very good substitute for oats, but is less
desirable by reason of its tendency to produce heat and fat. It is
therefore most useful in cold climates where more than the usual
amount of animal heat is required.

188. Feeding corn.—Corn may be fed whole, either shelled or
on the cob, or it may be crushed. It is usually given as a part
ration only.

189. Characteristics of corn.—Corn should be dry, hard, of
bright color, and free from dirt; when bitten into it should taste
sweet and have no distinct smell.

Heated, discolored, or moldy corn is unfit to use.

190. Weight of corn.—Seventy pounds of corn on the cob should
make 1 bushel or 56 pounds of shelled corn.

191. Kafir corn—Milo maize.—In emergencies, both these
grains may be fed the same as corn. Weight, 56 pounds to the
bushel.

192. Barley.—Barley is a very good horse feed, and may be used
as a substitute for oats. It may be fed whole, but is better crushed
or soaked in water for two or three hours before feeding. Weight, 48
pounds to the bushel.

193. Characteristics of barley.—Barley should be plump and
short, hard, with a thin wrinkled skin and small, fine, but not
shrunken ends. It should be of a pale golden yellow color, and
free from odor, dirt, and discolored grains.

194. Spelt or emmer.—This grain resembles barley and may
be used in the same way.

195. Rye.—Rye may be fed in emergencies in quantities not
exceeding 8 to 10 pounds a day.

196. Wheat.—Wheat is not a satisfactory food for horses, and
should be used only in cases of emergency. It is fed in quantities not exceeding 6 pounds daily.

197. Flour.—Flour may be fed to horses, but it should be made
into a sloppy gruel before giving.

198. Rice.—Unhusked rice, after the horses become accustomed to it, is a useful grain, and as much as 14 pounds may be fed daily. Only unhusked or unthrashed rice should be used.

199. Linseed meal (flaxseed meal, oil meal).—An excellent food for horses that have become run down in condition. It has a slightly laxative action, produces an oily skin and a sleek glossy coat, and may be given with other feed in quantities of from ½ to 1 pound daily.

200. Bran.—Bran is an excellent food for the horse. Fed once or twice a week in the form of a mash it proves a mild, beneficial laxative. When used continuously, the animal system becomes accustomed to it and the laxative property is less marked. Dry bran in small quantities is said to have a constipating effect.

201. Characteristics of bran.—Bran should be light in weight, dry, sweet, flaky, free from lumps and dirt, and sweet to the taste.

202. Bran mashes.—A bran mash is made by pouring boiling water on 2 or 3 pounds of bran in a bucket. A tablespoonful of salt may be added, and the whole covered up and set aside until sufficiently cool.

INDICATIONS OF DISEASE.

203. Loss of appetite.—Loss of appetite is usually one of the first indications of disease. It may, however, be due to overeating, excitement, or fatigue.

204. The pulse in disease.—Any deviation from the normal, strong, full, and regular pulse indicates an abnormal condition.

A rapid, full, bounding pulse is found in the first stages of fever.

A weak, small, and rapid pulse occurs in the later stages of fever and is an indication of great weakness.

A quick, feeble, fluttering pulse indicates the approach of death.

An abnormally slow pulse denotes disease or injury to the brain or spinal cord.

205. Breathing in disease.—Difficult or rapid breathing in animals at rest is a prominent symptom of disease of the respiratory organs; it may also be observed in some cases of flatulent colic.

206. Temperature in disease.—In fever or in diseases of an inflammatory nature the temperature of the body rises above the normal standard. In contagious diseases a rise of temperature often precedes any visible symptoms, a fact which is of great importance in detecting and weeding out suspected animals.

When in a locality where such diseases as surra, influenza, or contagious pneumonia are known to exist, early morning temperatures of all the animals of the organization should be taken regularly every day, or at least every other day. Any animal showing a temperature of 102° F., or over, should be isolated at once.

CARE OF THE SICK.

207. Nursing.—By nursing is meant the prompt and well-directed attention to the comforts and needs of the patient. Good nursing is therefore of the utmost importance in the care of the sick and injured.

208. The sick stall.—The first and most important point is to place the sick animal in a clean, light, well-ventilated box stall, free from drafts and located as far as possible from other animals. Clean bedding should be provided and the stall kept free from manure and moisture. If such a stall can not be obtained, a double stall, with the kicking bar removed and ropes or bars placed across the back of it, will answer the purpose. During cold seasons, paulins or horse covers may be hung in such a manner as to protect the patient from drafts, care being taken to allow sufficient air to enter this improvised stall.

Horses suffering from diseases of the nervous system, such as tetanus, require to be kept absolutely quiet, and must be removed as far as possible from all noise. It is best that only one man be allowed to attend them, as a change of attendants may cause excitement and thus increase the severity of the disease.

A horse suffering from colic requires a well bedded space sufficiently large to prevent injuring himself while rolling during the spasms of pain. In such cases a man should be constantly in attendance, as the animal may become cast and unable to get up without assistance.

In the field sick animals should be kept by themselves and made as comfortable as circumstances may permit.

209. Clothing.—Clothing, when required, should be provided according to the season. It should be light as well as warm, and should be changed, brushed, and aired at least once a day.

210. Bandaging for warmth.—When circumstances require it, the legs should be well hand-rubbed and wrapped in flannel bandages evenly and loosely applied. Bandages should be changed and the legs well rubbed twice daily.

211. Shoes.—Animals which are likely to remain on sick report for some time should have their shoes removed.

212. Feeding sick horses.—Only the choicest food, and food suitable to the requirements of each case, should be provided. The grain ration must be reduced, and the appetite tempted with daintily prepared food, such as fresh grass, bran mashes, carrots, or steamed oats. Green alfalfa, or cured alfalfa which has been soaked for an hour or two in clean water to which a small quantity of salt has been added, is usually eaten with great relish.

A lump of rock salt should be kept in the manger at all times.

Food should be given often and only in such quantities as the patient will readily eat. The feed should be placed within easy reach, and any portion left over should be at once removed and the feed box thoroughly cleaned—washed.

Food that is wet, such as bran mashes or steamed oats, soon sours in warm weather and gets cold or may freeze during the winter. If eaten in this condition it may cause diarrhea or colic.

Horses suffering from colic should have food withheld for at least 12 hours after all pain has disappeared, and then fed only in small quantities during the next 24 hours.

213. Watering sick horses.—A supply of fresh water should be kept constantly within reach and changed at least three times a day or oftener in warm weather.

214. Grooming sick horses.—Horses that are weak and depressed should not be worried with unnecessary grooming. Such animals should be carefully hand-rubbed or wisped at least once a day, and their eyes, nostrils, and docks should be wiped out with a sponge or soft cloth. The feet must also be cleaned.

Animals that are only slightly indisposed should be groomed in the usual way.

Animals with tetanus should not be cleaned at all.

215. Utensils to be kept clean.—Buckets, feed boxes, mangers, and all utensils used in or about the sick stall must be kept absolutely clean.

CARE OF THE INJURED.

216. Seriously injured animals.—When an animal is seriously injured and stands with difficulty, it should be placed in slings (par. 243, fig. 37) to partially support the weight of the body. For slinging, a single stall, having a level floor, free from bedding, is more suitable than a large one.

217. Slightly injured animals.—When an animal is but slightly injured there is no necessity of placing it in slings. An ordinary stall with a level floor is all that is required.

After an injury has been dressed the patient should be allowed to stand without being disturbed. If very lame and movement is painful, the quieter he is kept the more quickly will recovery take place.

218. Rest.—Absolute rest and perfect quiet are essential, and when secured they hasten the process of recovery without inflicting unnecessary pain.

219. Restraint of injured animals.—In some cases it becomes necessary to restrain the animal so that he can not injure himself by rubbing or biting the affected parts. This may be done by cross-tying (see par. 235), or by the use of the neck cradle (par. 233, fig. 30), or side rod (see par. 234, fig. 31).

220. Bandaging injured parts.—Bandages are used on the legs of injured animals to check bleeding, to protect the injured parts, and to support packs used in applying hot and cold lotions. Bandages should be adjusted evenly, and not so tight as to cause pain or obstruct the circulation.

221. Feeding, watering, and grooming of injured animals.—See paragraphs 211, 212, 213.

MISCELLANEOUS.

222. Feeding horses that bolt their feed.—Horses that eat rapidly and greedily are said to *bolt their feed*. To compel such animals to eat more slowly, let 1 pound of dry bran form a part of each feed, or place several large round stones in the feed box among the grain.

223. Feeding idle horses.—Horses which for any reason are compelled to stand idle for a day or more should have their grain ration reduced to 6 or 7 pounds a day, depending upon the condition of the horses, and 2 pounds of bran in the form of a mash should form a part of each daily ration.

224. Feeding thin horses and delicate feeders.—Such animals should be kept by themselves and fed a little at a time and often. The diet should be changed frequently, and should consist of grass, alfalfa, bran, either dry or in the form of a mash, linseed meal, steamed oats, and hay slightly damp and sprinkled with salt. A supply of fresh water should be kept constantly within reach.

225. Halter pulling.—Halter pullers may be secured by fastening ropes or chains across the stall behind them, or they may be turned loose in a box stall. The habit may be broken in the earlier stages by a slip noose about the flank, the rope being carried forward between the front legs, through the halter ring, and fastened securely to the manger or a post. To prevent injury, a folded sack or piece of cloth should be secured beneath the rope at the point where it passes over the back.

226. Windsucking and crib biting.—These are incurable vices which usually increase with age. Causes unknown. They are thought, however, to be a result of idleness, and to be learned by imitation. Keep such horses by themselves to prevent others from learning the habit. Place them in smoothly finished stalls without mangers or racks and feed off the floor.

227. Condition.—Condition is fitness for work. Horses that have been idle from injury or disease are not in condition, and should not be put to hard or fast work until they have received from one to three weeks' preparation in the way of gradually increasing exercise. Walking is the exercise which develops muscles; walking alternated with steady short trots, is the best method of getting horses in shape.

227½. Exhaustion.—Exhausted horses should receive a good stimulant (aromatic spirits of ammonia, nitrous ether, etc.), and their legs and body should be well rubbed and massaged. They should also be provided with a good bed. If on the march they should be unsaddled or unharnessed, a rest should be permitted and a drink of water provided, after which they may be taken slowly to camp. In hot weather put the animal in the shade and apply ice or cold water to the head. In cold weather blanket the body and bandage the legs. When rested, feed bran mashes, grass, hay, and steamed oats.

CHAPTER IV.

RESTRAINT AND CONTROL OF ANIMALS.

228. The object of restraint is to quiet or secure the animal in such a manner that it may neither injure itself nor those that are handling it. All experience demonstrates that animals which are most refractory and vicious under harsh and violent management will become reassured and tractable when treated with ordinary kindness and gentleness. Nervous and excitable animals especially should be dealt with quietly, so as to calm them and gain their confidence when they are about to be submitted to restraint and pain. Noise and excitement should be avoided as much as possible, and the preliminary stages of applying apparatus of restraint gone through steadily, intelligently, and with gentle hands and voice.

The apparatus should inconvenience or pain the animal as little as possible, and it ought to be readily applicable reliable when in

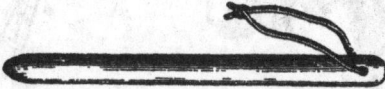

FIG. 28.—Twitch. (From Flemming's Operative Veterinary Surgery.)

use, and easily removed when no longer required. The respiration should be interfered with as little as possible. The horse and mule breathe only through the nostrils; therefore, these should be kept free and open. The trachea, chest, and flanks should not be pressed upon, as difficulty in respiration alone will cause violent struggling and may result in suffocation.

229. The kind of restraint to be used will generally depend not only upon the nature of the purpose for which it is intended, but also upon the disposition or temperament of the horse. The horse is secured in the standing position by the head or legs or both.

230. Securing the head.—The head is usually secured by means of a switch, blindfold, neck cradle, or side rod.

231. The twitch (fig. 28).—The twitch is a severe instrument of control, and should not be applied unless absolutely necessary. It is too frequently used on horses which could be more easily and humanely managed by gentleness, patience, and tact.

The ordinary twitch is a round piece of wood, from 1 to 5 feet in length, and 1½ to 2 inches in diameter, with a hole near one end through which a piece of cord is passed and tied in a loop sufficiently large to allow the closed fist to pass through easily.

The loop is passed over the upper lip, which is seized by the hand and drawn forward, care being taken to turn the edges of the lip in to prevent injury to the mucous membrane; the cord is then twisted by turning the stick until sufficient pressure is obtained, which is usually manifested by the closing of the animal's eyelids.

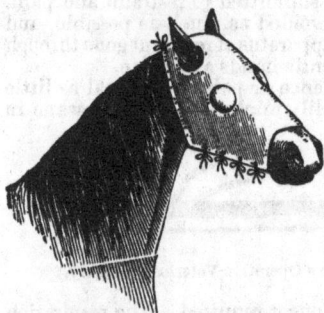

FIG. 29.—Blindfold. (From Flemming's Operative Veterinary Surgery.)

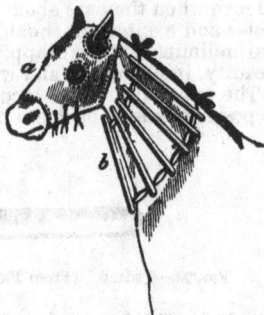

FIG 30.—Neck cradle. (From Flemming's Operative Veterinary Surgery.)

232. The blindfold (fig. 29).—Sudden deprivation of sight often so alarms or stupefies horses that they are rendered quite docile, or at least more manageable, while if really vicious they can not take advantage of a favorable opportunity to injure those around them.

Any nontransparent covering will exclude the vision; an empty grain sack, towel, or piece of cloth tied across the face from one side of the halter or head stall to the other, but the leather mule blind or the operating hood is best if available.

233. The neck cradle (fig. 30 *b*).—The neck cradle allows lateral and downward movements of the head to only a limited extent. This may be used to prevent the animal from biting and tearing his wounds, the dressings, or the blanket.

It is composed of from 8 to 12 round pieces of hardwood, about 1½ inches in diameter and about 18 inches in length, pierced at each end by a hole, through which a cord passes. These rods are kept 3 or 4 inches apart either by knots on the cords or by short pieces of wood perforated from end to end, and strung on the cord between the rods. The ends of the cords are tied on the upper border of the neck and so adjusted that the upper ends of the rods are just back of the lower jaw, the lower ends resting on the shoulder at the seat of the collar.

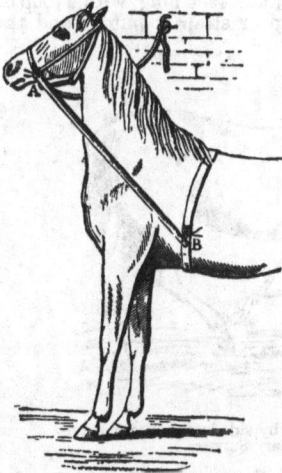

Fig. 31.—Side rod. (From Flemming's Operative Veterinary Surgery.)

234. The side rod (fig. 31).— The side rod is a round wooden rod, from 3½ to 4 feet in length, with a cord or small strap and buckle at each end. One end (A) is attached to the nose band of the halter, while the other (B) is fastened to a surcingle firmly secured around the body at the girth. The side rod is used to prevent the tearing of dressings or clothing with the teeth.

235. Cross tying.—Cross tying is useful in keepng an animal from lying down, and in preventing the tearing of dressings or clothing with the teeth.

It consists in tying the head in an elevated position with two tie ropes, one attached on either side of the halter to the rings in the nose band, and tied, one on either side of the stall, in such a manner as not to allow the nose to be lowered below the point of the shoulder. The food should be placed in a raised manger or rack.

236. Muzzles.—Muzzles should be constructed of leather or heavy woven wire, and should have a snap on either side for attachment to the side rings of the halter. They may be applied to vicious horses that bite, or to animals that have digestive diseases to prevent their taking food.   They are useful also to prevent animals from licking their wounds or tearing their dressings.

237. Securing a foreleg.—(*a*) With a rope or strap: A rope or a strap may be used to attach the pastern to the forearm.   The leg is well bent at the knee, and the rope or strap is attached to the pastern by means of a loop and then passed around the forearm and back to the pastern and tied.

A broad leather strap with a double loop and a strong buckle is to be preferred, as it is less likely to injure the leg.

(*b*) The side line: This is a rope about 20 feet long, with a loop or a hobble strap at one end.   The loop or strap is put around the

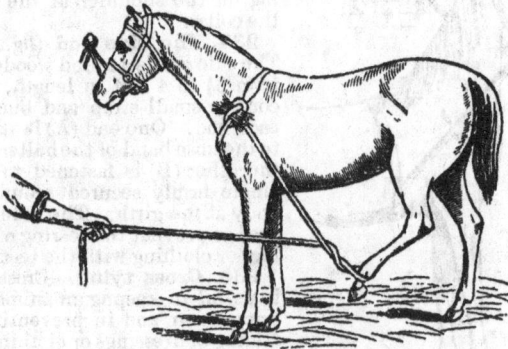

Fig. 32.—Securing a hind leg forward by side line. (From Flem-ming's Operative Veterinary Surgery.)

pastern of the limb to be raised, and the rope is passed over the horse's back to the opposite side, where it is held by an assistant after the leg has been lifted up and well flexed; or it is passed in front of the chest, around over the back to the same pastern, where it is tied, the weight and strain being thus thrown on the back.

The side line may also be used in securing the hind leg.

238. Securing a hind leg forward by side line, first method.— See figure 32.

239. Securing a hind leg forward by side line, second method.—See figure 33.

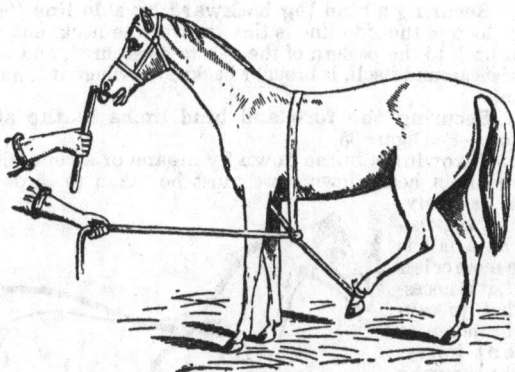

FIG. 33.—Securing a hind leg forward by side line. (From Flemming's Operative Veterinary Surgery.)

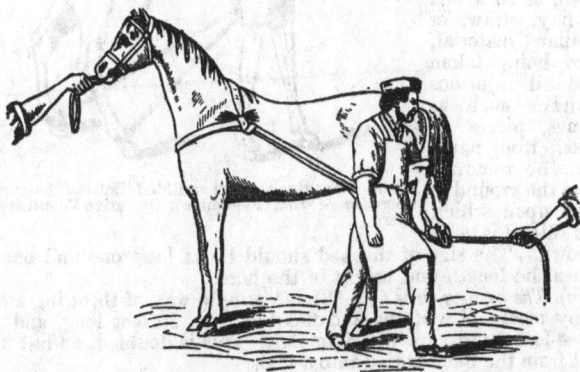

FIG. 34.—Securing a hind leg backward by side line. (From Flemming's Operative Veterinary Surgery)

240. Securing a hind leg backward by side line (fig. 34).—
A large loop of the side line is thrown over the neck, and the rope
carried back to the pastern of the foot to be secured, and by one or
two twists around itself, is brought backwards where it is held by an
assistant.

**241. Securing the fore and hind limbs in the standing
position.**—See figure 35.

242. Throwing a horse down by means of a rope (fig. 36).—
In throwing a horse down, care must be taken to throw him as
quickly, securely,
and safely as possi-
ble. As a fall is
always more or less
violent, it is neces-
sary that precau-
tions be taken to
prevent injury,
either by throwing
the horse on soft
ground, as on the
lawn, or on a bed
of hay, straw, or
similar material,
care being taken
that all injurious
bodies such as
stones, pieces of
wood, iron, nails,
etc., be removed
from the ground or
floor upon which
the animal is to be

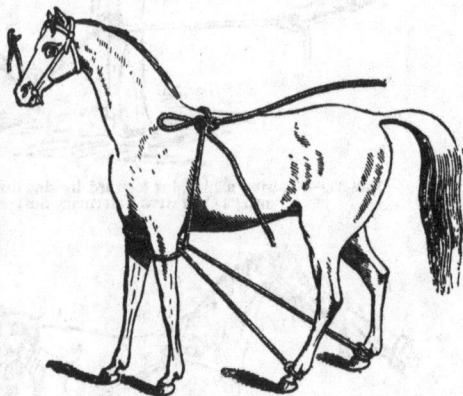

FIG. 35.—Securing the fore and hind limbs in the standing
position. (From Flemming's Operative Veterinary Surgery.)

thrown. The size of the bed should be at least one and one-half
times the length and height of the horse.

(a) *The casting rope* (fig. 36).—A simple way of throwing a horse
is by means of a strong and flexible rope, 30 feet long, and from
three-fourths to 1 inch in diameter. This is doubled, and at 2 or 3
feet from the bend is tied into a knot.

The loop thus formed is passed over the animal's head and the
rope adjusted as shown in figure 36. A strong man holds the horse's

head, on which there is a strong halter, and a twitch on the nose if necessary.

Two or three assistants pull, at a given signal or word, each rope backward, this draws the hind legs suddenly upward and forward, the animal then either falls or is easily pushed over on its side, when the ropes can be fastened to the loop around the neck by means of several half or double-half hitches, and the fore limbs secured to the hind ones by the same means.

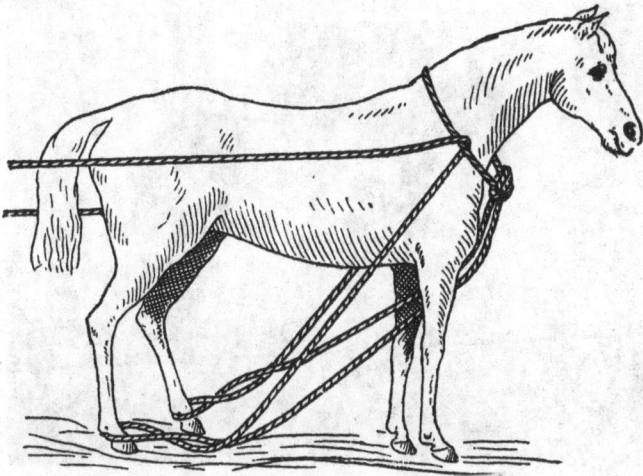

FIG. 36. The casting rope applied. (From Flemming's Operative Veterinary Surgery.)

As soon as the horse falls the man at the head places one knee on the neck and raises the horse's nose from the ground, turns it back toward the body and retains it in that position until the animal is released.

243. Slinging the horse (fig. 37).—When a horse is so severely injured as to stand with difficulty, or if it is desired to keep him in the standing position without allowing him to move about, the slings may be used. Before using, all parts should be carefully inspected

to make sure that they are strong enough to support the weight of the
animal. They must be so adjusted as to fit closely behind the
elbows in such a manner as to bear the weight of the body on the
chest and not on the abdomen. This position is maintained by the
use of the breast strap and breeching, which prevent the shifting of
the body girth. The slings must not be too tightly drawn; the
animal should stand squarely on his feet, and there should be just

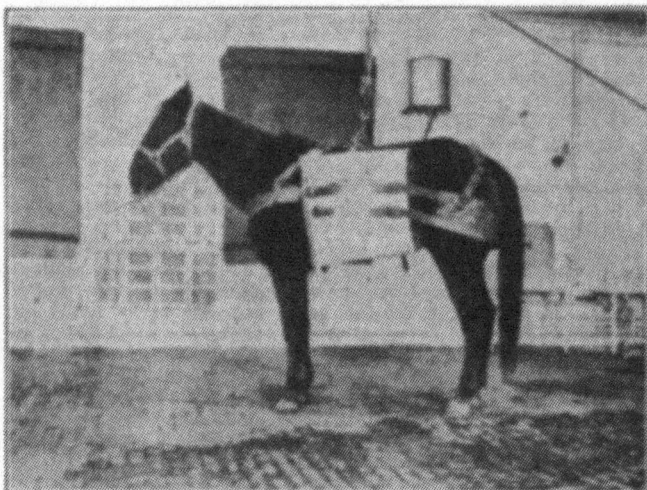

Fig. 37.—The horse in slings.

room enough between the front border of the body girth and the chest
to admit the insertion of two fingers

The slings are only intended to aid in standing. If the patient
refuses to bear weight on his legs and attempts to lie down, the stall
should be well bedded, the animal gently lowered to the floor, and
the slings removed.

The stall in which the slings are placed should be level, dry, and
free from bedding.

106233°—17——6

CHAPTER V.

ADMINISTRATION, ACTIONS, AND USES OF MEDICINES.

244. Administration of medicines.—Medicines may enter the body through any of the following channels: By the mouth; by the lungs and upper air passages; by the skin, externally; by the rectum; by the skin, hypodermically; by injection into a vein (intravenously)

245. By the mouth.—(*a*) In the form of powders, by placing the drug upon the tongue or in the food. When given in the food the powder should be mixed with the handful of wet bran or oats, for if placed in the dry oats the powder will sift through them to the bottom of the box where the animal will not get it; if it has a marked taste it should be well covered up in plenty of bran mash.

(*b*) In the form of a ball, made by rolling the drug in tissue paper or by putting it into a capsule.

To give a ball: The ball is held by the four fingers of the right hand. The left hand grasps the horse's tongue, carefully pulls it out, and turns it upward in the right interdental space so that it opens the mouth. With the right hand the ball is carried well back into the mouth and dropped at the root of the tongue. When the right hand is withdrawn, the left hand carries the tongue to the middle of the mouth and releases it. When the tongue is released the ball is carried backward into the pharynx and swallowed.

(*c*) In the form of a drench, by first elevating the head and then slowly pouring the liquid into the mouth. This is a difficult procedure at times, and in all cases needs to be done carefully and slowly, pouring only a little into the mouth at a time in order to avoid wasting the medicine and to prevent choking the animal. If the animal should cough the head must be lowered at once to allow the liquid which has entered the larynx to be expelled.

(*d*) By injecting the liquid into the back of the mouth by means of a syringe.

246. By the lungs and upper air passages.—Medicines are brought in contact with the mucous lining of the respiratory tract by inhalation. Inhalations are given by placing a bucket containing hot water or scalded bran, to which 1 ounce of turpentine, carbolic acid, or creolin has been added, in the bottom of a gunny sack. The

horse's nose is then inserted into the top of the sack where it is held
from 20 to 30 minutes. Or hot bricks may be placed in a pail and
tar or other medicine poured upon them and the animal allowed to
inhale the vapor. Liquids should under no consideration be injected
or poured into the nostrils.

247. By the skin.—Medicines are applied to the skin for their
local action only: (a) To destroy parasites; (b) for their antiseptic
action; (c) for their soothing or stimulating effect; (d) for their blistering action.

248. By the rectum.—Medicines may be given by the rectum
when the animal is unable to swallow; also to destroy worms in the
rectum, and to cause evacuation of the bowel. For the latter purpose warm water is most useful.

249. By the skin, hypodermically.—Medicines are given under
the skin, in concentrated form (alkaloids), when prompt action is
desired. Such medicines are to be used only as directed by the
veterinarian.

250. By injection into a vein.—Medicines are administered
into a vein when rapid action is required. This method is used only
by veterinarians.

WEIGHTS AND MEASURES.

251. Weights.
          60 grains (gr.)....................1 dram (ℨ).
          8 drams.........................1 ounce (℥).
          16 ounces........................1 pound (lb.).
252. Liquid measure.
          60 minims (min.).................1 fluid dram (f ℨ).
          8 fluid drams...................1 fluid ounce (f ℥).
          16 fluid ounces..................1 pint (Oi).
          32 fluid ounces..................1 quart (Oii).
          4 quarts........................1 gallon (Ci).

253. Solutions are liquid preparations containing substances
which readily dissolve.

(a) A saturated solution is made by adding to a liquid all of a
drug that the liquid will dissolve

(b) To make—

One per cent solution of creolin, add 1 part creolin to 99 parts water.
Two per cent solution of creolin, add 2 parts creolin to 98 parts
water.

Three per cent solution of creolin, add 3 parts creolin to 97 parts water.

Four per cent solution of creolin, add 4 parts creolin to 96 parts water.

Five per cent solution of creolin, add 5 parts creolin to 95 parts water.

Ten per cent solution of creolin, add 10 parts creolin to 90 parts water.

Twenty per cent solution of creolin, add 20 parts creolin to 80 parts water.

Fifty per cent solution of creolin, add 50 parts creolin to 50 parts water.

Water and creolin are used above merely as example. Other fluids—alcohol, ether, glycerine, etc.—are also used in making solutions.

(c) To make—

One per cent solution of a solid drug, add 1 part of the solid to 100 parts of water.

Two per cent solution of a solid drug, add 2 parts of the solid to 100 parts of water.

Three per cent solution of a solid drug, add 3 parts of the solid to 100 parts of water.

Four per cent solution of a solid drug, add 4 parts of the solid to 100 parts of water.

Five per cent solution of a solid drug, add 5 parts of the solid to 100 parts water.

Ten per cent solution of a solid drug, add 10 parts of the solid to 100 parts water.

254. Mixtures are liquid preparations containing substances which do not dissolve.

255. Liquid measure—approximate value.

A drop ....1 minim.
A teaspoonful ....1 dram.
A tablespoonful ....4 drams (½ ounce).
Ordnance tin cup, old style ....28 ounces.
Ordnance tin cup, new style ....22 ounces.

One minim always equals one-sixtieth part of a dram; a drop does not, for drops of various liquids differ in size and weight.

256. Metric measures.

1 c. c. stands for 1 cubic centimeter and equals 16 minims.

4 c. c. equal 1 dram by measure.

30 c. c. equal 1 ounce

500 c. c. approximately equal 1 pint.

1,000 c. c. approximately equal 1 quart.

257. Dry measure—approximate value.—An ordnance spoon holds approximately 1 ounce of—

Salt,

Zinc sulphate.

Lead acetate.

Potassium nitrate.

Potassium permanganate, etc., when heaping full.

An ordnance spoon holds approximately 2 drams of—

Gentian.

Fenugreek.

Ginger.

Nux vomica, etc.

ACTIONS AND USES OF MEDICINES.

258. Antiseptics.—Agents, used on or in the body in the treatment of wounds or diseases, which prevent the growth and development of germs. Ex.: Carbonic acid, bichloride of mercury, iodine, creolin, etc.

259. Anesthetics.—Agents that produce loss of the sense of touch or pain. Ex.: Chloroform and ether.

260. Astringents.—Agents which contract tissues and check secretions. Ex.: Alum, zinc, tannic acid, etc.

261. Anodynes.—Agents which relieve pain. Ex. Opium, belladonna, cannabis indica.

262. Antispasmodics.—Agents which prevent or allay spasmodic contraction of voluntary or involuntary muscles. Ex.: Belladonna, cannabis americana.

263. Alteratives.—Agents which reestablish the healthy functions of the body. Ex : Potassium nitrate and potassium iodide.

264. Carminatives.—Agents which aid in the expulsion of gas from the stomach and intestines. Ex.: Ginger, turpentine, aromatic spirits of ammonia.

265. Caustics.—Agents which destroy tissue by burning. Ex.: Copper sulphate, lunar caustic (silver nitrate).

266. Cholagogues.—Agents which promote secretion of bile. Ex.: Calomel, aloes.

267. Disinfectants.—Agents which destroy the germs that cause infectious diseases. Ex.: Chloride of lime, carbolic acid, creolin, formalin.

268. Deodorants.—Agents which disguise or destroy odors. Ex.: Creolin, carbolic acid.

269. Diuretics.—Agents which increase the excretion of urine. Ex.: Nitrate of potash, turpentine, nitrous ether.

270. Expectorants.—Agents which act upon the mucous membranes of the respiratory organs and favor the removal of their secretions. Ex : Ammonia chloride, tar, turpentine.

271. Febrifuges (antipyretics).—Agents which reduce fever. Ex.: Nitrous ether, quinine, cold water.

272. Laxatives.—Mild cathartics. Ex.: Small doses of oil, bran mash, green foods.

273. Purgatives (cathartics).—Agents which empty the bowels. Ex.: Aloes, salts, and linseed oil.

274. Parasiticides.—Agents which kill animal and vegetable parasites infesting the skin. Ex.: Carbolic acid, creolin, salicylic acid.

275. Stomachics.—Agents which promote digestion. Ex.: Gentian, ginger, fenugreek.

276. Styptics.—Agents which check hemorrhage. Ex.: Tincture of iron.

277. Stimulants.—Agents which promptly but temporarily increase nervous vigor. Ex.: Alcohol, aromatic spirits of ammonia, ether.

278. Sedatives.—Agents which soothe the nervous system. Ex.: Bromide of potassium, cannabis indica.

279. Tonics.—Agents which gradually but permanently improve the general health and increase vigor. Ex.: Iron, sulphate, gentian, nux vomica.

280. Vesicants (blisters).—Agents which cause inflammation of the skin with a discharge of serum under the epidermis. Ex.: Cantharides, biniodide of mercury.

Blistering.—Clip the hair, and brush away the dirt from the part to be blistered, then apply the blister and rub briskly for from 5 to 20 minutes, the amount of rubbing depending on the thickness of the skin and the effect desired. The longer the rubbing is kept up the more severe will be the effect. In thin-skinned horses, rubbing for five minutes is usually sufficient. The animal should then be controlled by cross tying or tying the head up short to prevent him from biting, rubbing, or lying on the blistered area. The tail must be tied up if within reach of the blister. The blister should be left on for 24 hours and then washed off and the parts kept clean and well oiled to prevent cracking of the skin. Blisters should not be applied to the back of joints or to any acutely inflamed parts.

281. Vermicides.—Agents which kill intestinal worms. Ex.: Turpentine, copper sulphate, iron sulphate.

282. Vermifuges.—Agents which remove intestinal worms by purgation. Ex.: Aloes, linseed oil.

MEDICINES.

283. Acetanilid.—Antiseptic. Used externally as a dusting powder, alone or in combination with other drugs.

284. Acid, arsenious (arsenic).—Irritant, caustic poison. It is sometimes given as a tonic in the form of Fowler's solution in ½ to 1 ounce doses.

285. Acid, boracic (boric acid).—Nonirritant antiseptic. Used in all strengths up to a saturated solution as a mild soothing antiseptic in diseases of the eyes, and as a wet or dry dressing for wounds. Also in the form of an ointment for burns, etc., strength 10 per cent. Used alone or in combination with other drugs.

286. Acid, carbolic (phenol).—A caustic, disinfectant, and antiseptic. Pure carbolic occurs in crystals which may be dissolved by heat and the addition of glycerin, alcohol, or water. Carbolic acid is a powerful poison and is readily absorbed from raw surfaces, hence must not be used too freely in strong solutions. A 5 per cent solution may be used to disinfect the unbroken skin, but on raw surfaces, a 2 per cent solution is sufficiently strong. When applied externally in full strength it burns the skin and causes it to turn white. This burning action may be stopped by the application of alcohol. In poisoning, alcohol, brandy, or whisky should be given.

287. Acid, salicylic.—A useful antiseptic, but irritating to the tissues and but slightly soluble in water. A saturated alcoholic solution is of value in the treatment of indolent sores and ulcers.

288. Acid, tannic.—Astringent. Dose ½ to 2 drams. Useful internally in the treatment of diarrhea and dysentery, given alone or in combination with other drugs. Externally it is used to check bleeding from raw surfaces; in solution, in alcohol or witch-hazel, it may be used to harden tender shoulders. It is also useful in the form of an ointment, 1 to 4, for scratches, etc.

289. Alcohol.—Stimulant and antiseptic. Dose 2 to 4 ounces in a pint of water every four to six hours, as required. Of great value in the treatment of debilitating diseases.

290. Aloes, Barbados.—Purgative. Dose 6 to 8 drams. This is a slow but powerful-acting cathartic, taking about 24 hours to operate. Of value whenever an active purge is desired. May be given in the form of a ball or in solution in hot water. It should not be given when there is great weakness, a tendency to diarrhea, or in respiratory diseases Ginger is generally given with aloes to overcome the griping which it causes.

Drams.

Aloes 6–8
Ginger...: 1–2

Make into a ball.

291. Alum.—Astringent and styptic Used externally in the treatment of thrush. In a 2 per cent solution it is valuable as a wash for sore mouths.

292. Ammonia, aromatic spirits.—Stimulant and carminative. Dose 1 to 2 ounces diluted with 1 pint of water. Of great value in exhaustion, and in the treatment of colics.

293. Ammonia, aqua (solution of ammonia).—Used externally only and in the form of stimulating liniments.

Parts.

Aqua ammonia...................................... 1
Turpentine.. 1
Olive oil... 2

Shake well before using.

Of value to relieve the pain caused by insect stings, i e , bees, wasps, etc.

294. Ammonia, chloride of.—Expectorant. Dose, 2 to 4 drams. Useful in all irritable conditions of the respiratory mucous membranes.

295. Belladonna, fluid extract of.—Antispasmodic and anodyne. Dose, ½ to 2 drams. Used internally in colics to relieve pain and spasms. Useful in eye lotions to relieve pain and to dilate the pupil. In the treatment of painful affections of the eye the following is of value:

Zinc sulphate.............................grains.. 20
Belladonna, fluid extract..................dram.. 1

Water to make 4 ounces.

Drop a few drops into the eye twice a day with a dropper.

296. Camphor, gum.—Antispasmodic, stimulant, expectorant, antiseptic. Dose, 1 to 2 drams It is useful in the treatment of diarrhea. Externally it is used in liniments for its stimulating and anodyne actions. A useful preparation known as *soap liniment* is made as follows.

	Parts
Castile soap	10
Camphor, gum	5
Alcohol	70
Water	15

297. Cannabis indica or cannabis americana, fluid extract of.—Anodyne, antispasmodic. Dose, 2 to 4 drams Very much used in the treatment of colics, as it relieves pain without causing constipation; also of value in the treatment of tetanus to control the muscular spasms.

298. Cantharides, powdered (Spanish fly).—Vesicant. Used only for its blistering effect, made up in an ointment with cosmoline in the strength of 1 part cantharides to 4 or 6 parts of cosmoline. Prepare by rubbing the ingredients together with a spatula.

299. Charcoal.—A mild antiseptic and deodorant. Used as a dry dressing for foul-smelling wounds, either alone or in combination with other drugs.

300. Chloroform.—Antispasmodic, anodyne, and carminative. Dose, 1 to 2 drams. Local anesthetic when rubbed into the skin and a general anesthetic when inhaled.

301. Creolin.—Disinfectant, antiseptic, parasiticide, and deodorant. Used principally as an antiseptic in 1 to 2 per cent solutions; also in the same strength or up to 5 per cent to destroy parasites of the skin. Useful in the form of an ointment; strength, 5 to 10 per cent. To disinfect nail wounds in the foot apply creolin full strength on cotton or oakum. A good ointment for parasitic skin diseases is made as follows:

	Parts
Acetanilid	10
Creolin	5
Cosmoline	20

Melt the cosmoline and while cooling add the other ingredients. Creolin is also used internally as a vermifuge, 1 ounce in a quart of water, given on an empty stomach. To kill rectal worms, give 1 ounce creolin in a quart of water as an injection.

302. Chloro-naphtholeum (Kreso).—Action same as creolin, but not so useful, being more oily and less refined. Principally used as a disinfectant

303. Collodion.—Used as a protective dressing for wounds. When painted on the skin it rapidly dries and leaves a thin protective coating. The skin must be dry or the collodion will not adhere.

304. Cosmoline (petrolatum, vaseline).—Used as a base for ointments and as a soothing agent applied to blistered or abraded surfaces.

305. Digitalis, fluid extract of.—A dangerous poison

306. Ether, spirits nitrous (sweet spirits of niter)—Stimulant, antispasmodic, and diuretic. Dose, 1 to 2 ounces. This is one of the most generally useful drugs we have. Used in the treatment of fevers, especially those accompanied by weakness. An excellent remedy in the treatment of colic, combined with belladonna or cannabis indica.

307. Ether, sulphuric.—Stimulant, antispasmodic, carminative, and, when inhaled, anesthetic. Dose, 1 to 2 ounces, well diluted. Useful in the treatment of thumps. Given in colics, especially flatulent colics, to diminish the production of gas and cause its expulsion. It may be given alone or with other drugs.

308. Flaxseed meal (linseed meal).—A laxative food, and an excellent poultice material.

309. Formalin.—Antiseptic, disinfectant, and deodorant. Used externally only. It is very irritating and should not be used stronger than 1 dram to a quart of water (approximately one two-hundredth) for ordinary purposes.

310. Genetian, powdered.—Stomachic, and bitter tonic. Dose $\frac{1}{2}$ to 1 ounce. It increases the secretions of the stomach and intestines and improves the appetite. Usually combined with other drugs.

311. Gentian, fluid extract.—Action, uses, and dose, same as the powdered drug. May be given diluted, when the animal will not take the powder in the feed.

312. Ginger.—Stomachic and carminative. Dose, 2 drams to 1 ounce. Used in indigestion accompanied by flatulency. Also in combination with purgatives to hasten their action and lessen the griping caused by them.

313. Glycerine.—Used as a base in the same manner as cosmoline. Used internally in cough mixtures to moisten and soothe the throat   The following is a useful cough remedy

```
Fluid extract belladonna ................drams..   4
Nitrous ether............................ounces..   2
Glycerine................................do....   2
Water to make ...........................do....   8
```

Mix and give one-half ounce three times daily.

314. Iodine crystals.—Alterative, absorbent, and antiseptic. Seldom used internally. Used externally, iodine is a powerful antiseptic. The tincture is made by dissolving 1 ounce of the crystals in a pint of alcohol. A good solution for external use is made as follows:

```
Iodine .....................ounce..   1 ⎫ Lugol's
Potassium iodide.............do....   3 ⎬ solution.
Water .......................pint..   1 ⎭
```

Either the tincture or the solution is valuable in the treatment of wounds, sores, ulcers, curbs, splints, enlarged tendons, etc. For such purposes it is applied once or twice daily with a small cotton swab.

315. Iodoform. Antiseptic.—It contains more than 90 per cent of iodine and is a valuable agent in the treatment of wounds. It may be used alone or in combination with other drugs, as:

Acetanilid and boric acid, equal parts.
Iodoform sufficient to give a light yellow color.

316. Iron, tincture, chloride of.—Styptic and tonic. A valuable agent for building up the system and enriching the blood. Useful during recovery from debilitating diseases. Dose, 1 to 2 ounces, well diluted.

317. Iron, sulphate of.—Tonic, astringent, and vermicide. Dose, $\frac{1}{2}$ to 1 dram. Used internally as a tonic and to destroy worms. Used externally as an astringent dusting powder.

318. Lead, acetate of sugar (sugar of lead).—Astringent. Used externally in the form of *white lotion*, for its cooling and soothing action in the treatment of sprains, bruises, itching skin diseases, cuts, burns, and scratches. All local conditions with heat, pain, and swelling are benefited by its use. *White lotion* is made as follows:

```
Lead acetate..............................ounce..   1
Zinc sulphate.............................do....   1
Water to make.............................quart..   1
```

Shake well and apply several times daily.

319. Lime, chloride of.—Disinfectant and deodorant. Must be fresh and kept in sealed jars. Used 6 ounces to the gallon of water to disinfect stables.

320. Liquor cresolis (solution of cresol).—Antiseptic and disinfectant. Used externally in 1 to 2 per cent solutions. It is a powerful antiseptic and much less poisonous than carbolic acid. It froms a soapy solution and is a very efficient cleaning agent.

321. Lunar caustic (silver nitrate).—Caustic. Used for the removal of excessive granulations (proud flesh) and warts and to stimulate slow healing ulcers.

322. Mercury, bichloride of (corrosive sublimate).—Antiseptic and disinfectant. Put up in tablets containing 7½ grains of mercury. One tablet to a pint of water makes a 1-1000 solution, the strength most commonly used in the treatment of wounds. If in bulk, used 7½ grains of bichloride of mercury to a pint of water, and add 7½ grains of ammonium chloride or table salt to insure solution of the mercury.

323. Mercury, mild chloride of (calomel).—Cholagogue, purgative, antiseptic, and drying. Dose, ½ to 1 dram. Frequently combined with aloes to make the physic ball:

Calomel	drams	½–1
Aloes	do	4–6
Ginger	do	1

Water to make a ball.

Used externally as a dry dressing in the treatment of thrush.

324. Mercury, biniodide of (red iodide).—Used as a blistering agent in the treatment of spavin, splints, ringbone, sidebone, thickened tendons, etc.

A mercury blister is prepared as follows:

Parts.

Biniodide of mercury	1
Cosmoline or lard	5–6

Mix and rub together thoroughly.

325. Nux vomica, fluid extract of.—A nerve stimulant and tonic. Dose, 1 to 2 drams. Very useful in the treatment of debilitating diseases. Usually given with other drugs, gentian, iron sulphate, etc.

326. Nux vomica, powdered.—Action and dose the same as the fluid extract. These drugs must not be given for more than five or six days at a time, as poisoning may result.

327. Oil, linseed.—Laxative. Dose, 1 to 2 pints. Much used in the treatment of colics. The *raw oil* should always be used.

328. Oil, olive.—Laxative. Dose, 1 to 2 pints. Principally used in making oily solutions for external use and as a soothing application in irritable conditions of the skin.

329. Oil, turpentine.—Stimulant, diuretic, antispasmodic, antiseptic, carminative, expectorant, and vermicide. Dose, 1 to 3 ounces, well diluted with oil. This is a most useful drug and of great value in the treatment of colics, especially flatulent colic. As a vermicide a single large dose, 2 to 4 ounces, is given in a pint of linseed oil, on an empty stomach. Used externally in stimulating liniments and to disinfect nail wounds. Given as an inhalation in respiratory diseases, 1 to 2 ounces to a pail of boiling water.

330. Opium, tincture of (laudanum).—Anodyne, and antispasmodic. Dose, 1 to 2 ounces. It checks secretion from mucous membranes and is of value in the treatment of diarrhea and dysentery.

331. Opium, powdered.—Action same as tincture. Dose 1 to 2 drams.

332. Potassium arsenate, solution of (Fowler's solution).—Alterative and tonic   Dose, $\frac{1}{2}$ to 1 ounce

333. Potassium bromide.—Nerve sedative. Dose, 1 to 2 ounces. Used to allay nervous excitability. In tetanus it is given in very large doses, 2 to 8 ounces

334. Potassium iodide.—Alterative, diuretic, and expectorant. Dose, 2 to 4 drams.

335. Potassium nitrate (saltpeter).—Alterative, febrifuge, diuretic. Dose, 2 to 4 drams. Internally much used in the treatment of fevers. In the treatment of laminitis it is used in large doses, 2 to 4 ounces, two or three times daily. Externally it is used as a cooling lotion in the treatment of sprains and bruises:

Potassium nitrate..........................ounces..	5
Ammonia chloride..........................do....	5
Water...pint..	1

Mix and keep the affected parts saturated with the solution.

336. Potassium permanganate.—Antiseptic, disinfectant, and deodorant. Used externally as an antiseptic in the treatment of wounds, 1 to 2 drams to the pint of water. Full strength it is mildly caustic.

337. Quinine, sulphate of.—Tonic, stomachic, antiseptic, and febrifuge. Dose, ½ to 1 dram three times daily. Used in the treatment of all febrile (fever) diseases.

338. Soap, castile.—A cleaning agent. Used in removing grease and dirt from the skin surrounding the margins of wounds. Should not be applied to raw surfaces. Also used in making soap liniment.

339. Sodium bicarbonate.—Stomachic. Dose, 2 to 8 drams. Used externally to allay itching and the pain of slight burns, ½ to 1 ounce to a pint of water. Used internally in chronic indigestion.

340. Sulphur.—Parasiticide. Used in the form of an ointment in the treatment of skin diseases such as mange and eczema:

	Parts.
Sulphur	1
Lard	4

Apply twice a day.

341. Tar, pine.—Antiseptic, stimulant, expectorant, and parasiticide. Dose, 2 to 4 drams. Used as a protective dressing in the treatment of corns and punctured wounds of the foot. Also in the treatment of skin diseases. A good application is made as follows:

	Ounces.
Tincture iodine	2
Sulphur	1
Oil of tar	4
Olive or linseed oil to make 1 pint.	

Mix. Shake well before applying.

First thoroughly cleanse skin, and, when dry, rub the mixture in well and leave on for several days. Wash off and repeat if necessary.

342. Witch hazel.—Astringent. Used externally as a cooling application to reduce swelling and relieve pain.

343. Zinc, sulphate of.—Antiseptic and astringent. Used externally in the form of *white lotion,* for the treatment of bruises, collar sores, sore shoulders, saddle sores, etc.

344. Zinc oxide.—Mildly astringent and antiseptic. Used as a dry dressing for wounds, either alone or in combination with other drugs: Zinc oxide, boric acid, and acetanilid, equal parts.

Also used as an ointment in the treatment of abrasions and scratches.

	Parts.
Zinc oxide	1
Cosmoline	4

345. Bandages.

Flannel.—Use chiefly on the legs for warmth, support, protection, and the retention of dressings.

Cotton.—Used for the retention of dressings and the protection of wounds.

346. Dressings.

Absorbent cotton.—Used as a substitute for sponges in the cleansing of wounds; to make packs by soaking it in medicinal solutions; and to retain dry dressings in contact with the surfaces of wounds.

Antiseptic gauze.—A light, loosely woven variety of cloth, which has been saturated with an antiseptic and dried. Used as a covering for wounds. Gauze must be kept clean and the part that is to come in contact with the wound should never be touched with the fingers or hands.

Oakum.—Prepared fiber from old ropes. Used principally in packing horses' feet. It may also be used as a substitute for sponges, and, in the absence of cotton and gauze, as a covering for wounds.

347. Packs.—Packs are made by soaking cotton, gauze, oakum, or similar material in hot or cold medicinal solutions, after which they are applied to the part with a bandage.

348. Poultices.—Poultices are preparations for the local application of heat and moisture. They are made usually of flaxseed meal and bran, but other substances, such as oatmeal and bread, may be used. The material from which they are to be made is stirred up in hot water until thick and pasty. This mass is then spread on a piece of sacking or cloth of any kind and applied, while hot, directly to the part and held in place by means of bandages or other appliances. When poultices are intended for use on wounds, such as punctures of the foot, etc., from 2 to 4 drams of carbolic acid or creolin should be added to the mass to render it antiseptic.

Poultices are most useful about the feet. They should be changed twice daily and immersed in hot water every hour to keep them fresh and to prevent drying. Their application should not be continued for more than three or four days at a time.

349. The field medicine chest.—The following supplies are ordinarily sufficient for a troop of cavalry for one month, and are intended for use in the field when no veterinarian accompanies the troops. They should be carefully and tightly packed in a well made box with a hinged lid, hasp, staple, and padlock. The drugs should be kept in glass stoppered bottles, if obtainable, and all bottles and boxes should be plainly labeled with name and dose of contents and the labels well pasted on. Use the oakum for packing the bottles, and as it becomes used up for other purposes replace it with sacking or other suitable material. To prevent the wasting of medicine in the field, great care should be taken not to make up at any one time more than is actually needed.

Basin, granite, 1-quart...............................	1
Drenching bottle, pint, leather covered............	1
Twitch, short, to fit in box.........................	1
Farrier's instrument pocket case, in canvas or leather cover....................................	1
Eye dropper...	1
Graduate glass, 2-ounce.............................	1
Syringe, metal or hard rubber, 2 to 4 ounces capacity...	1
Extra corks, assorted sizes................dozen..	1
Ammonia, aromatic spirits of.............ounces..	8
Ammonia liniment.........................do....	8
Belladonna, fluid extract of................do....	1
Bandages, cotton.........................dozen..	1
Bandages, flannel.........................do....	⅓
Bichloride of mercury tablets.............ounces..	2
Cotton, absorbent.........................do....	16
Cannabis Indica or Americana............do....	4
Creolin or Kreso..........................do....	16
Drying powder............................do....	8
Ether, nitrous............................do....	8
Eye lotion, saturated solution of boracic acid, ounces...	4
Gauze, antiseptic........................package..	1
Iodine, tincture of.......................ounces..	8
Lead acetate..............................do....	8
Oakum....................................pounds..	2
Potassium nitrate.........................ounces..	8
Potassium permanganate..................do....	2
Soap, castile.............................pounds..	1½
Tar, pine.................................do....	1
Zinc sulphate.............................ounces..	8
Zinc ointment, in 4-ounce tins.............do....	8
Silk for sutures and needles in packet case.	

CHAPTER VI.

WOUNDS AND THEIR TREATMENT.

Wounds.

350. A wound is an injury to any part of the body involving a separation of the tissues of the affected part.

Wounds are classified as *incised, lacerated, punctured, bruised,* and *gunshot*.

Incised wounds are clean cuts made by a sharp instrument.

Lacerated wounds are injuries in which the tissues are more or less torn. They are made by blunt objects, such as hooks and the teeth of horses and mules.

Punctured wounds are made by pointed objects, such as nails, splinters, thorns, and the prongs of forks and rakes.

Bruised wounds are injuries in which the skin is not broken, such as are caused by falls, kicks, the bumping of various parts of the body against blunt objects, and by pressure from the saddle and collar.

Gunshot wounds are those made by bullets or pieces of shell.

Dressings.

351. A dressing is a form of local treatment producing a continuous action. It consists in the methodical application, upon the surface of a wound, of medical substances, and the use of such protective agents as gauze, cotton, or oakum, suitably arranged and held in position by bandages or other means.

Wounds are not healed by treatment. The object of treatment is to keep the injured parts clean and protected, and *nature* repairs them. *Cleanliness* is, therefore, the all-important principle in their handling. Not only should the wound itself be clean but also the dressings, the instruments, and the vessels in which these are contained.

The person doing the dressing should have his *hands thoroughly clean,* and should procure in a *clean* basin or bucket an *antiseptic solution*, and a sufficient quantity of clean cotton, gauze, or oakum He should also make ready the necessary instruments, as follows:

Instruments.—Scissors, knife, forceps, probe, syringe, and a needle and some thread, if required; all to be clean and placed in a tray or a basin and immersed in any good antiseptic solution, except *bichloride* of *mercury*, which will corrode them.

GENERAL TREATMENT OF WOUNDS.

352. Stop the bleeding (hemorrhage).—If bleeding is profuse and from large vessels, the first step is to stop the flow of blood, This may be done by grasping the bleeding vessel or vessels with the forceps and tying them with a piece of silk, string, horsehair, or any suitable material which may be at hand.

If the vessel can not be tied, a thick pad made of cotton, gauze, oakum, or clean cloth may be made and bandaged tightly over the wound. This arrangement is called a *compress* and should not be kept on for more than three or four hours, after which it must be removed and a clean dressing with less pressure applied.

If the wound be in a location which will not permit bandaging, the bleeding may be stopped by packing it tightly with cotton or gauze held in place by stitches in the skin drawn tightly over the packing.

Slight hemorrhages, such as follow injuries to the small vessels and capillaries, may be checked by baths of cold water or by compresses of cotton or oakum, either dry or soaked in a solution of *tincture* of *chloride* of *iron.*

353. Clean the wound and remove all foreign bodies.—When the bleeding has stopped, cut the hair from the edges of the wound and remove all dirt, clots of blood, splinters, and foreign bodies of every kind. This may be done by carefully syringing the parts with clean warm water, or a warm antiseptic solution. Foreign bodies may be removed with the forceps or by passing small pieces of cotton soaked in an antiseptic solution gently over the surface of the wound. These pieces of cotton must be thrown away after using and not put back in the solution. The object of this is to keep the solution and the rest of the material clean. Wounds that are clean and dry should *not* be washed.

354. Apply an antiseptic.—*Tincture* of *iodine, iodoform, boracic acid,* or a solution of *carbolic acid, creolin,* or *bichloride* of *mercury.*

355. Close the wound.—Sutures and bandages are used for this purpose, but no wound that has been dirty must ever be entirely closed.

Sutures as a rule may be dispensed with entirely. They may occasionally be used in parts where there is little flesh, such as around the forehead, eyelids, and nose. They are less useful in fleshy parts, because the movements of the muscles and the swelling resulting from the inflammation of the injured tissues cause them to pull out. Again, sutures must not be used when the edges of the wound are badly torn.

In applying sutures, the borders of the wound must be brought together in their natural position, care being taken not to allow the edges of the skin to curl inward. The thread, with the aid of a needle, is passed through the skin at one side of the wound and out at the other. The sutures should be from one-fourth to one-half an inch from each edge, about three-fourths of an inch apart, and their depth should be about equal to their distance from the edge of the wound. They should be drawn just tight enough to bring the edges of the skin together. As a rule, they should be removed in about eight days.

356. Drainage.—In all wounds drainage is necessary for the removal of serum and pus that would otherwise accumulate in them. The escape of such material must be provided for at the lowest part of the wound. If the wound be a vertical (upright) one, this may be accomplished by leaving out a stitch at the bottom. In horizontal wounds (wounds running lengthwise with the body), a small vertical opening must be made below the line of stitches.

357. Dressings.—Wounds that have been sutured and also wounds that are to be treated without suturing, should be dried carefully with dry gauze or cotton, painted with tincture of iodine, or dusted with an antiseptic powder, covered with dry gauze or cotton and a bandage applied. Or, cotton soaked in an antiseptic solution may be put on and held in position by a bandage, care being taken to avoid undue pressure.

If the location of the wound will not permit bandaging, the injured parts may be painted with tincture of iodine or dusted with an antiseptic powder, and covered with a clean piece of cloth or gunny sack, the inside of which may be lined with a piece of gauze large enough to cover the wound.

358. Rest and restraint.—This will depend entirely upon the nature and extent of the wound. If the injury be slight, the animal may continue at work; otherwise he may be kept in a box stall, cross-tied, or placed in slings.

359. After care.—All wounds should be kept dry, and dressings should be changed only often enough to keep the wound clean. As little washing as possible should be done, and the parts should be sopped instead of rubbed. After cleaning and drying a new dressing must be applied.

360. Flies.—The healing of wounds that can not be covered is sometimes retarded by the presence of flies. Such wounds should be painted once or twice daily with either of the following preparations:

A.

Creolin, ½ ounce.
Oil of tar, 1 ounce.
Oil, olive, 10 ounces.
Mix.

B.

Carbolic acid, 3 ounces.
Camphor, 8 ounces.
Mix.

361. Maggots (screw worms).—Wounds sometimes get fly-blown and maggots appear. Their presence is recognized by a thin bloody discharge from the wound and the red, angry appearance of its edges. If the bottom of the wound is carefully examined, movement of the worms may be seen.

Treatment.—With forceps, pick out all the worms that are visible and wipe out the cavity with a swab of cotton that has been saturated with a solution of *carbolic acid* 1 to 5. Or *turpentine* 1 part and *olive oil* 3 parts may be used in the same way.

362. Excessive granulations (proud flesh).—In sluggish, slow-healing wounds, small rounded, fleshy masses are often formed, which protrude beyond the edges of the wound. These fleshy masses are called *excessive granulations* or *proud flesh*.

Treatment.—The growths must be kept down by the use of astringents, or caustics, such as alum, nitrate of silver, or sulphate of copper or zinc.

SPECIAL TREATMENT OF WOUNDS.

363. Incised wounds.—See "General treatment of wounds."

Lacerated wounds.—Trim away all torn and ragged edges and treat as directed under general treatment of wounds. If pockets are formed, provide drainage.

Punctured wounds—Punctured wounds, except those around joints, should be carefully probed to ascertain if any foreign bodies are present. If so, they must be removed, and, if the wound runs in a downward direction, an opening should be made a little lower down to allow for drainage. The wound is then swabbed out with a strip of gauze that has been saturated with *tincture of iodine*, or it may be syringed out very carefully with an *antiseptic* solution, care being taken not to force the stream in a downward direction. After cleaning the interior, a dusting powder should be applied to the surface.

364. Punctured wounds or joints and tendon sheaths.—Punctures of the synovial membrane of joints or tendons, which allow the synovia to escape, are always serious and often result in permanent disability or death of the animal. The conditions are commonly known as *open joint* and *open bursa*, respectively,

Treatment —Do not probe unless a foreign body is known to be present, as the introduction of the probe, even though clean, may injure the delicate structures of the joint or tendon sheath.

Remove the hair; cleanse the parts, but do not use the syringe; paint the opening of the wound with *tincture of iodine*, apply a *biniodide of mercury* blister, and cover with gauze and a bandage. Place the animal in slings or a cross-tie; clean the wound daily, if required; paint with *tincture of iodine*, and rebandage. If the wound be a large one, omit the blister and treat with antiseptics.

Feed laxative foods and keep fresh, cool water before the animal at all times.

BRUISED WOUNDS (CONTUSIONS) AND ABRASIONS.

365. Under this heading are considered *sore backs* and *sore shoulders*, etc.; otherwise known as *chafes* and *galls* of the back or shoulders or any part that comes in contact with the saddle, harness, or equipment.

366. Sore backs.—This term includes all injuries produced by the pressing or rubbing of any part of the saddle or saddle equipment against the skin and its underlying tissues, the nature and severity of such injuries depending upon the amount of pressure and the length of its duration.

Sway-backed horses, roach-backed horses, horses with bulging barrels or barrels tapering upward and backward, or horses with abnormally high or abnormally low withers, are more liable to such injuries than others.

Causes.—1. Faulty placing of the saddle, i. e., too far forward or too far back.   2. Improper folding of the blanket; blanket wrinkled,

dirty, and containing sand, burrs, splinters, thorns, etc., in its folds.
3. Improper adjustment of the equipment, and unequal distribution
of weight. 4. Drawing the cincha too tight and improper adjustment of the cincha and quarter straps. 5. Poor riding, i. e., lounging
in the saddle and shifting from one side to the other. 6. Improper
adjustment of the stirrup strap, i. e., too long or too short or unequal
in length. 7. Long continuous work under the saddle. 8. Pro-
fused sweating and rain.

Symptoms —Hard, hot, painful swellings, appearing usually
within an hour after unsaddling. These lesions are best detected
by passing the hand over the back, when swelling and tenderness
may be discovered.

As a result of continuous pressure the skin often becomes bloodless,
dies, dries up, and gets hard and leatherlike. This dead piece of
skin is called a *sitfast*. Later, if the animal is continued in use, the
skin sloughs off, leaving raw sores of various sizes and depths. Injuries to the withers or along the top of the spine, frequently terminate in *abscesses*. (See Abscess.)

Treatment.—Ascertain and remove the cause, if possible. In fresh
cases, apply cold irrigations or baths with gentle hand rubbing.
This is to be followed by the application of cold in the form of packs
saturated and kept wet with cold water and held gently in position
by means of a surcingle or bandage. The pad may be of oakum,
or it may be made by folding a gunny sack three or four times. Ice
packs or cold lotions may also be used.

Injuries to the *withers* and *ridge* of the *spine* should be irrigated
or bathed with cold water, but without pressure and without massage.

When sitfasts appear, apply warm baths or warm linseed poultices
until the dead skin becomes loose; it is then removed with the forceps
and a knife, after which the injury is treated with *tincture* of *iodine*
or an *antiseptic powder*.

Slight *galls*, *chafes*, or *abrasions* (spots rubbed bare) are treated
with *white lotion*, *zinc oxide ointment*, powdered *boracic acid*, or a
solution of *tannic acid* 1 ounce in a pint of *witchhazel* or *alcohol*.

Prevention.—Adjust carefully and properly the saddle, the blanket,
and the equipment; keep the blanket clean, dry, and free from foreign material; sit properly in the saddle, and dismount frequently
and walk.

After long marches, loosen the cincha slightly and leave the saddle
on for from 30 minutes to an hour after dismounting. Where an
injury has occurred, the blood vessels are compressed and almost
bloodless. If pressure be now suddenly and completely removed,

blood is vigorously forced into the paralyzed vessels and may rupture their walls. On the other hand, if the saddle be allowed to remain for some time in position, circulation may be gradually restored without injury.

367. Injuries from packsaddles and aparejos.—The causes, nature, and treatment of these injuries are the same as those produced by the riding saddle.

368. Sore shoulders.

Causes.—Dirty, ill-fitting, and improperly made collars; excessive weight of the pole, causing pressure on the top of the base of the neck; improper adjustment of the hames or trace plates; unequal length of traces; working with head drawn to one side; long continuous work in the harness; rough roads, and poor driving.

Treatment.—Same as for sore backs (par. 366).

Prevention.—Fit the collars properly and keep them clean; keep the mane closely trimmed at the base of the neck; adjust the pole chains properly, and drive with care.

369. Bruises of the limbs.

Causes.—Kicks, falls, treads, and, in draft animals, blows from the pole.

Treatment.—Cold irrigations and cold packs. When the inflammation is reduced apply tincture of iodine or a blister, if required

GUNSHOT WOUNDS.

370. Gunshot wounds are those made by bullets or pieces of shell.

Treatment.—Do *not* probe for bullets unless they can be distinctly felt through the skin. Leave them where they are and they will either become embedded in the tissues or expelled by the process of suppuration (formation of pus).

The tract of the bullet must *not* be irrigated nor should any attempt be made to explore its depths. The point of entrance, and that of exit, too, if there be one, should be treated locally with antiseptics, preferably *tincture* of *iodine*.

The animal should be watched daily for the formation of an abscess which may develop and disclose the location of the bullet.

SEROUS SACS.

371. By the term *serous sac* is meant a collection of serum, a straw-colored, sometimes bloody, watery fluid, under the skin.

Causes.—Blows and bruises, particularly about the buttocks.

Symptoms.—A uniformly soft, painless, fluctuating swelling, varying in size from that of an egg to a man's head. They often resemble windgalls and hernias (ruptures of the abdominal wall), from which they must be carefully differentiated.

Treatment.—Bathe twice a day for a week with cold water, and follow each bath by applications of *white lotion.* If, at the end of this time the swelling has not disappeared, apply *tincture of iodine* or a blister. About two months are required to effect a cure. Opening the enlargement is inadvisable and should be left to the veterinarian. The animal may be worked, except when the swelling is so located as to be injured by the saddle or harness.

SUPPURATION—ABSCESS.

372. Suppuration.—By this term is meant the formation and discharge of pus (matter).

An *abscess* is a local collection of pus in the tissues of any part of the body. From eight days to two or three weeks' time is usually required for its development.

Causes.—It is usually the result of an inflammation caused by an injury. Abscesses also frequently occur in the course of certain diseases, such as distemper, pneumonia, and pharyngitis.

Symptons.—Heat, pain, and swelling in the injured part. The swelling is at first small and hard. It gradually increases in size, however, and finally becomes soft and elevated in the middle into a prominent hairless spot. This is called *pointing* or *coming to a head.* In a few days after pointing begins the abscess opens and its contents (pus) escape.

Treatment.—Small abscesses in the early stages may be scattered by the application of cold packs or *tincture of iodine.* The best results, however, are usually obtained by the use of warm baths or warm *linseed poultices.* When the swelling becomes soft in the center, it should be opened at its lowest point, using a sharp instrument to cut through the skin and a blunt one to enlarge the opening and prolong it into the cavity of the abscess. A sharp instruments must not be deeply inserted into the cavity, as large blood vessels may be injured and fatal bleeding follow.

After opening, the cavity must be flushed once or twice daily with an antiseptic solution until pus ceases to flow.

Abscesses, like serous sacs, sometimes resemble windgalls and hernias from which they must be carefully differentiated, as opening a hernia would be fatal.

BURNS AND SCALDS.

373. Treatment.—Bathe or tie up the parts with any mild antiseptic solution, or dust the surface with *borac acid* or *flour* and cover with cotton and a bandage. If sloughing occurs, treat as an ordinary wound.

INJURIES RECEIVING SPECIAL NAMES.

374. Capped elbow (shoe boil).
Causes.—A bruise at the point of the elbow produced by lying upon a hard unbedded floor.
Symptoms.—A hot, painful swelling at the point of the elbow.
Treatment.—Cold irrigations and *white lotion* baths. After the inflammation has been reduced, apply *tincture of iodine* daily or blister. If an abscess forms and the swelling bursts, syringe out daily with an antiseptic solution. Cross-tie the animal during treatment. Operative measures must be left to the veterinarian.
Prevention.—Keep the stall floor level and give plenty of bedding.

375. Capped hock (fig. 38).
Causes.—A bruise to the point of the hock caused by lying upon hard, unbedded floors, and by kicking against the stall or other hard objects.
Symptoms.—A hot painful swelling at the point of the hock.
Treatment.—Same as for capped elbow.
Prevention.—If due to kicking in the stall, pad the heel posts with gunny sacks and straw. If due to lying on a hard floor, provide a good bed

FIG. 38, 5.—Capped hock.

376. Fistulous withers (fig 39) — An abscess in the vicinity of the withers having a chronic discharge of pus from one or more openings. It may involve the soft structures only, or it may extend to the bones.
Causes.—Bruises, usually from the saddle or collar
Symptoms and treatment.—See abscesses, paragraph 372.

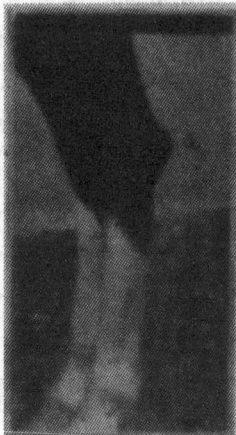

377. Poll Evil (fig. 40).—An abscess in the region of the poll.

Causes.—Bruises caused by the animal striking the poll against some overhead object, or by pressure due to pulling back on the halter.

Symptoms and treatment —See abscesses, paragraph 372

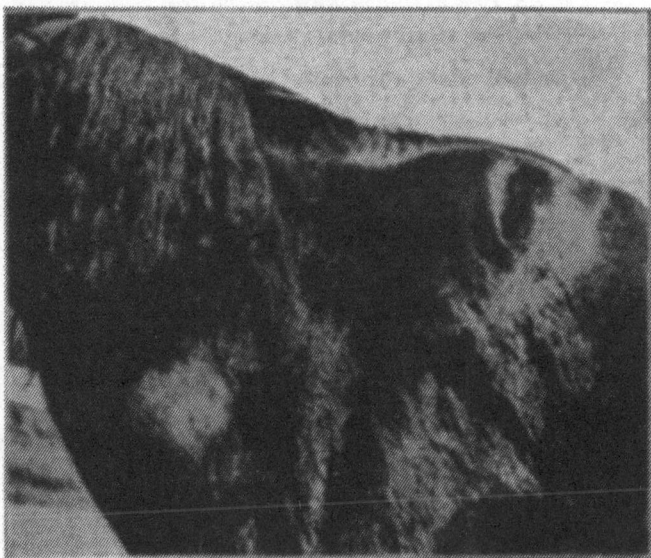

Fig. 39.—Fistulous withers.

378. Rope burns.—Abrasions or lacerations usually at the back of the hind-pasterns

Causes.—Getting the foot over the halter shank, picket line, or lariat. It is generally the result of leaving the halter shank too long in tying.

Symptoms.—The injury may be a simple chafe of the skin or it may involve the underlying tendons and ligaments.

Treatment.—Trim away all torn and ragged edges, clean the wound thoroughly and apply an antiseptic. See paragraphs 347, 354, 357,

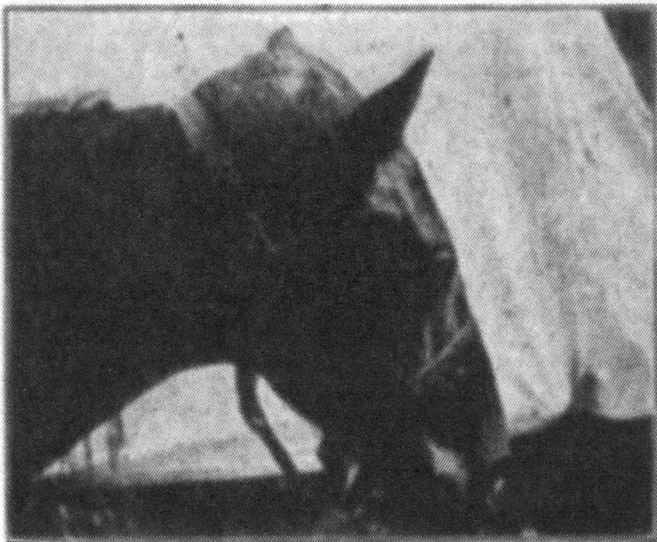

FIG. 40.—Poll evil.

358, and 359. Should the parts at any time become dry, hard, and painful, they may be softened by daily applications of *zinc oxide ointment* or *creolin* and *olive oil* (creolin ½ ounce, olice oil 4½ ounces).

INFLAMMATION.

379. Inflammation.—A condition into which the tissues of the body enter as a result of an injury.

Symptoms.—Pain, heat, swelling, and redness (invisible in dark skin and in skin covered with hair), all of which occur as the result of an increased flow of blood to the injured part.

Treatment.—Bathe or irrigate the inflamed area several times daily with cold water. When the parts will admit it, cold packs may be applied.

CHAPTER VII.

DETECTION OF LAMENESS—DISEASES OF BONE.

DETECTION OF LAMENESS.

380. Lameness.—Lameness is any irregularity in the gait.

381. Classification of lameness.—Lameness is divided into two classes

(a) *Swinging-leg lameness*, which is shown by a shortened stride and more or less dragging of the leg. Seen in diseased and injured muscles.

(b) *Supporting-leg lameness*, shown when the leg supports the weight of the body. This form occurs in diseases and injuries of bones, tendons, ligaments, and the foot.

382. Severe lameness is readily recognized, even when the animal is at rest. Distinct symptoms, such as pointing or frequently raising the injured limb, are usually seen, the animal's instinct leading him to place the affected part in a position to relieve the pain.

383. Examination for lameness.—In making an examination for lameness, the animal, having free use of his head, should be led at a slow trot toward and from the observer. Too short a hold on the halter shank prevents free play of the muscles concerned in locomotion.

In examining the lame limb, place it in its natural position and inspect its various parts both with the hand and eye, comparing them carefully with those of the sound leg for the purpose of detecting differences in shape, size, temperature, and sensitiveness to touch and pressure.

In all cases examine the foot thoroughly and carefully, removing the shoe if necessary. Heat, pain, and swelling are valuable guides in the detection of lameness. The *hoof tester* or pinchers, carefully and gently employed, is useful in locating injuries of the foot.

384. Lame in one fore leg.—When lame in one fore leg, the right one, for instance, the head nods (drops) more or less when weight is put on the left fore leg, while the head jerks up at the moment the right leg (the lame one) is placed upon the ground Hence, the head of the lame animal always nods when the foot of the sound leg is placed on the ground.

107

385. Lame in both fore legs.—Should there be lameness in both forelegs, the action is stilty (stiff); the natural, elastic stride is wanting; the steps are shortened, and the feet are kept close to the ground. The hind legs are invariably picked up higher than usual, the shoulders appear stiff, and the head is carried rather high, while the lumbar region is arched.

386. Lame in one hind leg.—Lameness behind is detected by trotting the horse from the observer, the croup being the part to be watched, since it drops with the sound leg and rises with the lame one.

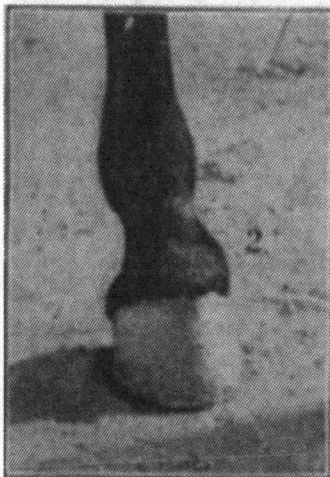

FIG. 41.—Ringbone.

387. Lame in both hind legs.—When lame in both hind legs, the stride is shortened and awkward; the fore legs are kept back of the vertical line, and are apt to be raised higher than usual while the head is lowered. Backing is difficult. It is almost impossible to keep the animal at a trot when it is lame in more than one leg.

Horses lame in both fore or both hind legs show a waddling gait behind, often mistaken for lameness in the lumbar region. This peculiar motion is simply due to the fact that the hind legs are unduly advanced under the body for their own relief or that of the front legs.

Close attention should be paid to the animal's action as he turns while being trotted to and from the observer, as at this moment—that is, while he turns—any hitch becomes visible, as, for instance, in spavin or stringhalt lameness.

DISEASES OF BONE.

388. Ringbone (fig. 41).—A ringbone is a bony enlargement occurring in the region of the long and short pastern bones. It occurs more frequently in the front legs than in the hind ones.

Causes.—Sprains, bruises, hard and fast work, and penetrating wounds involving the periosteum; improper shoeing, such as cutting the toe too short or leaving the heels too high, or leaving one side of the hoof wall higher than the other.

Symptoms.—Lameness, which may disappear with exercise, is usually the first symptom observed. Later, there appears a hard, painless swelling, over which the skin is freely moveable.

Treatment.—Remove the shoe and level the foot. Use cold baths and cold packs for a week, then apply a *biniodide of mercury* blister. Keep the animal in a level stall and give perfect rest for four to six weeks.

389. Side bone (fig. 42).—Side bone is a condition in which the cartilages of the foot have changed to bone. The disease is most frequently seen in heavy draft horses and in draft and pack mules. The front feet are affected more often than the hind ones, and the outer cartilage suffers more frequently than the inner one.

Causes.—Concussion produced by fast work on hard roads; allowing the feet to become dry and hard; lack of frog pressure; mechanical injuries, such as treads and similar wounds; and improper shoeing, i. e., leaving the heel too high or the use of high heel calks.

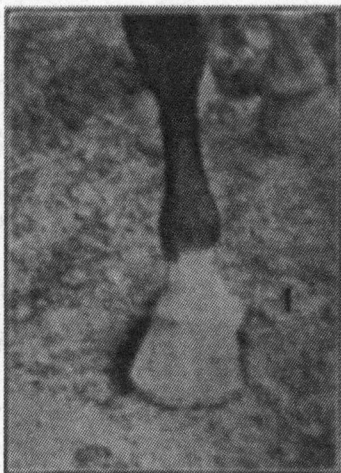

FIG. 42.—Sidebone.

Symptoms.—A hard, unyielding condition of the cartilages of the foot, with or without lameness.

Treatment.—This is necessary only when the animal is lame. In such cases remove the shoe, level the foot, and stand the horse in cold water for several hours a day, or apply a swab around the coronet and keep it wet with cold water. As soon as the inflammation has disappeared, apply a blister of *biniodide of mercury* over the part and keep the animal quiet in a level stall for three weeks.

390. Spavin (fig. 43) —Spavin is a disease affecting the bones of the hock joint and usually appears as a bony enlargement on the inner and lower part of the hock.

Causes.—Violent strains in rearing, jumping, pulling, or galloping, and severe rapid work, especially under the saddle. *Tied-in hocks* and *sickle-shaped hocks* are more likely to suffer than those that are broad and well developed.

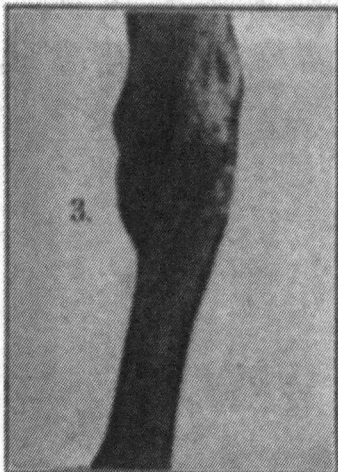

FIG. 43.—Spavin.

Symptoms.—The development of spavin is usually accompanied by lameness, which, in the earlier stages of the disease, is noticed only when the animal is first moved after a rest, at which time the toe is generally placed on the ground first, the heel not being brought down until the step is nearly completed. The bony enlargement may be present when the lameness appears, or it may not develop for several weeks thereafter.

Treatment.—The same as that prescribed for ringbone (par. 388).

391. Splints (fig. 44).— Splints are bony enlargements, usually situated between the inner splint bone and the cannon bone. They seldom occur on the hind leg.

Causes —Fast work on hard roads; improper shoeing favoring interfering and unequal distribution of weight on the leg.

Symptoms —In the early stages there is slight swelling, increased heat, pain on pressure, and more or less thickening. Lameness may or may not be present. When present, it disappears in the later stages and the swelling becomes hard.

Treatment —Necessary only when the animal is lame. If due to improper shoeing, remove the shoe and level the foot. Shower the part daily with cold water and follow each shower with a white lotion pack. When the inflammation has disappeared, apply a blister of *biniodide of mercury* and keep the animal quiet in a level stall for three weeks.

DISLOCATIONS.

392. A dislocation is the displacement or separation of the parts of a joint.

393. Dislocation of the patella (stifled).—A displacement of the patella from the end of the femur. The displacement may be upward or outward.

Causes.—Falls, slipping when trying to get up, and stepping down from an elevated position to the ground or floor below. It occurs sometimes as a result of weakness after or during the course of debilitating diseases.

Symptoms.—The displacement may be stationary, or the patella may slip in and out with every step. In the former, the leg is rigidly extended backward, the horse, even with assistance, being unable to bend the leg or carry it forward

Treatment.—Reduce the dislocation. By suddenly moving the animal backward the bone may return to its normal position. This failing, a rope is placed around the pastern and the leg drawn forward

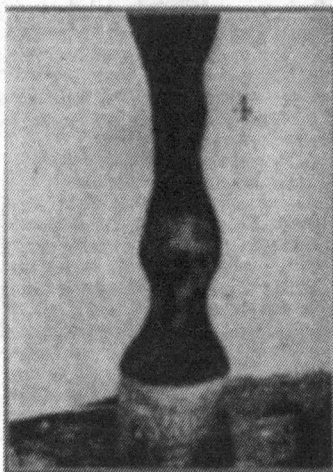

FIG. 44 —Splint.

and upward by an assistant, at the same time the operator presses the patella forward and inward with both hands. As the bone goes into place a clicking sound may be heard, and the animal at once regains control of the leg.

If the joint be painful and swollen, shower with cold water and bathe with white lotion until the inflammation is reduced, then apply a cantharides blister and give four weeks rest.

Should the dislocation recur, a rope should be fastened to the pastern and attached to a collar about the animal's neck. The rope should be drawn just tight enough to prevent the animal from extending his leg to the rear but allowing him to stand on it. The rope is kept on until the effect of the blister has passed away.

FRACTURES

394. A fracture is a break in a bone A fracture may occur in any part of the bony framework. The bones of the limbs, however, are more likely to suffer than those of other parts of the body.

A *simple fracture* is one in which the bone is broken into but two parts, the skin remaining unbroken

A *compound fracture* is one in which the broken ends of the bones protrude through the skin.

A fracture may also be complete or incomplete. An incomplete fracture is one in which the bone is not entirely broken across.

Causes —Falls, kicks, blows, or any form of mechanical violence.

395. Fracture of the bones of the limbs.

Symptoms.—Great and suddenly appearing lameness; excessive mobility; crepitation (a crackling or grating sound made by the rubbing together of the broken ends of the bone); and inability to bear weight on the injured limb. The animal usually evinces great pain and marked swelling occurs within a few hours.

Treatment.—Complete fractures are usually incurable and the animal should be destroyed to terminate suffering.

In incomplete fractures, or when such a fracture is suspected, the animal must be relieved from work and kept from lying down for a month, either by being cross-tied or placed in a sling.

396. Fracture of the lower jaw.—This refers to a chipping or splintering of the bone by the bit or the curb chain.

Causes.—Rough handling of severe bits and tight curb chains, and the use of chains or ropes passed through the mouth and around the jaw.

Symptoms.—The animal fights the bit and resists any attempt to handle the mouth. The mucous membrane covering the bone is swollen, hot, and painful, with perhaps a small fragment of bone sticking through it. In many cases the covering of the bone is entirely torn away. Suppuration occurs in a few days and the wound emits a very foul odor.

Similar injuries sometimes occur on the lower margin of the bone at the seat of the curb chain.

Treatment —Clean the part thoroughly and remove all fragments of bone   Tincture of iodine or a solution composed of *camphor gum* 8 ounces and *carbolic acid* 3 ounces is then carefully applied to the bottom of the wound by means of a very small cotton swab.   All particles of food must be removed and the dressing repeated daily until healing occurs.

CHAPTER VIII.

DISEASES AND INJURIES OF MUSCLES, TENDONS, AND LIGAMENTS.

SPRAINS.

397. Sprains are injuries due to excessive exertion. They affect muscles, tendons, and ligaments, the fibers of which are stretched or torn, causing inflammation, sometimes followed by contraction and, in muscles, atrophy (wasting away).

398. Sprains of the muscles.—Muscle sprains occur in various parts of the trunk and limbs, and are due to slips or falls. When sprained, the muscle becomes swollen, hot, and painful and loses its power of contraction. Later, it sometimes atrophies. Owing to the loss of function, the condition resembles paralysis, but in paralysis there is no heat, pain, or swelling.

399. Sprains of the flexor tendons (fig. 45).—The tendons at the back of the cannon are frequently injured, especially those of the fore legs.

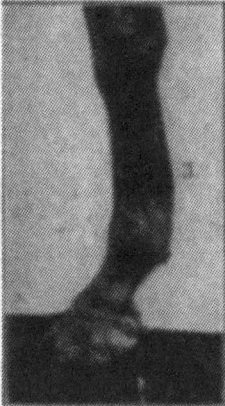

FIG. 45 —Sprained tendons.

Causes.—Long toes and low heels; violent efforts and sudden checks, as in jumping; and long-continued exertion in which the muscles tire, thereby increasing the strain on the tendons.

Symptoms.—Lameness, corresponding in degree with the severity of the injury; swelling, usually most prominent at the middle third of the cannon; heat and sensitiveness to touch.

Treatment —See paragraph 407.

400. Sprain of the suspensory ligament.

Causes.—Sudden violent efforts and long-continued exertion.

Symptoms.—Lameness. Heat, pain, and swelling in the region between the cannon bone and the tendon of the deep flexor of the foot, the swelling usually being most pronounced just above the fetlock.

Treatment.—See paragraph 407.

401. Sprain of the plantar ligament (Curb. fig. 46).

Causes.—Violent efforts at rearing, pulling, and jumping. Usually seen in horses with weak, narrow, overbent hocks.

Symptoms.—A firm swelling at the back and lower part of the hock, about 4 inches below its point, giving the region a curved appearance when viewed from the side. Lameness is rare.

Treatment.—When lameness is absent, treatment is usually unnecessary. If the swelling is painful and hot, treat as prescribed under general treatment of sprains. (Par. 407.)

402. Sprains of the hock, fetlock, and pastern joints.

Causes.—Violent exertion, slips, stepping on stones, traveling over rough, uneven ground.

Symptoms.—Lameness, accompanied by heat, pain on pressure, and swelling.

Treatment.—See paragraph 407.

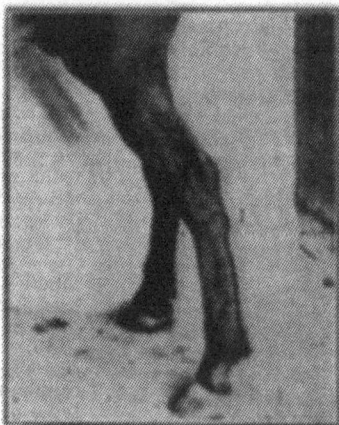

FIG 46.—Curb.

BURSAL AND SYNOVIAL ENLARGEMENTS.

403. Under this heading are described *bog spavin, thoroughpin,* and *windgalls* (wind puffs) of the fetlock. These enlargements are chronic nonsensitive conditions which rarely cause lameness.

404. Bog spavin.—A distention of the joint capsule of the hock, due to the presence of an abnormal amount of synovia, which causes the capsule to bulge outward and forward.

Causes.—Long continued hard work, particularly at jumping, pulling, and galloping.

Symptoms.—A soft puffy swelling situated in front and a little to the inside of the hock. Acute inflammation and lameness are rare.

Treatment.—Not usually necessary. If the parts are hot and painful, give rest and reduce the inflammation by cold irrigations. After a week of this treatment, apply *tincture of iodine* once a day for 10 days. This failing, a *cantharides blister* should be used.

405. Thoroughpin.—A condition usually associated with bog spavin.

Causes.—Same as bog spavin.

Symptoms.—A soft fluctuating swelling at the upper and back part of the hock, between the point of the hock and the lower end of the tibia.

Treatment.—Seldom required. See "Bog spavin."

406. Windgalls (windpuffs) of the fetlock.—A distention of the synovial bursae of the flexor tendons at the back of the fetlock joint.

Symptoms.—Soft puffy enlargements about the back part of the fetlock.

Causes and treatment —See "Bog spavin."

TREATMENT OF SPRAINS.

407. Treatment of sprains.—Rest Remove the shoes, level the feet, and place the animal in a level, well bedded box stall. (See pars. 216 to 221)

Bathe or shower the injured part for one-half hour twice a day with cold water and follow each bath with packs of *white lotion* (half strength) or cold water; or a lotion composed of *witch hazel* 1 pint, *lead acetate* 1 ounce, water 1 quart may be applied. Continue this treatment for one week, then use warm baths followed by warm packs or *soap liniment*. If, after the inflammation is reduced, the parts still remain swollen, apply *tincture of iodine* once a day for 10 days. This failing, apply the following blister and repeat in two weeks, if necessary:

```
Cantharides...................................dram.. 1
Biniodide of mercury.........................do..... 1
Cosmoline or lard............................do.... 6
```

Mix well.

In chronic sprains of the flexor tendons, shoe with short heel calks or thicken the branches of the shoe, or shorten the toe and leave the heels and quarters long.

CHAPTER IX.

DISEASES OF THE DIGESTIVE SYSTEM.

DISEASES OF THE MOUTH.

408. Injuries to the mouth.—These consist of lacerations of the membrane lining the lips, cheeks, and tongue.

Causes.—Blows; coarse, rough food materials; faulty teeth, and foreign substances, such as splinters, pieces of glass, and irritating plants in the forage. The tongue is sometimes torn by the bit and by rough handling in examining the mouth. In halter pullers it may be severely bitten.

Symptoms.—Slobbering; difficult and painful mastication; and laceration, heat, swelling, and redness of the injured parts

Treatment.—Remove the cause. Flush out the mouth twice a day with a solution of *potassium permanganate*, ½ dram to a quart of water, or *alum*, ½ ounce to a quart of water, or *creolin*, 2 drams in a quart of water may be used in the same way.

DISEASES OF THE TEETH.

409. Irregular wearing of the teeth.

Causes.—Abnormal inequality in the width of the upper and lower jaws. The upper jaw being the wider, the inner edges of the lower molars and the outer edges of the upper ones sometimes become abnormally long and sharp (sharp teeth). These sharp points frequently injure the cheeks and tongue.

The milk molars are sometimes not promptly shed, their remnants remaining as caps on the crowns of the permanent teeth.

In *undershot* and in *overshot* (parrot mouth) the teeth do not wear on each other, the result being that those receiving little or no wear become excessively long and injure the soft structures and bone with which they come in contact.

In old animals, due to unequal hardness of opposing teeth, the molars may become uneven in length, the harder ones sometimes wearing away the opposite ones and projecting into and injuring the soft tissues and bone at their roots.

Symptoms —Slobbering; difficult mastication; holding the head to one side while eating or drinking; dropping balls of partly chewed food from the mouth (quidding), and retaining food in the mouth for some time after eating.

Treatment —A dental operation is required.

410. Decay of the teeth.—Confined almost exclusively to the molars.

Causes.—Injuries, such as splitting of the tooth or the breaking away of the outer covering (enamel).

Symptoms.—An offensive odor about the mouth; slobbering; slow, painful, and difficult mastication; holding the head to one side while eating or drinking; dropping food from the mouth, and a collection of decomposing food around the diseased tooth. The decayed tooth has an offensive smell and may be broken, split, or shorter than the surrounding ones. If it be an upper one, there may be a discharge from the nostril of the same side.

Treatment —The diseased tooth must be removed. This is a difficult and dangerous operation, which only a veterinarian can perform.

DISEASES OF THE THROAT.

411. Choke.—An obstruction of the throat with a foreign body.

Causes.—Hurried attempts at swallowing oats, bran (dry), or pieces of carrots, apples, etc., before they have been properly masticated. Choke may also result from giving balls that are too large or of improper shape.

Symptoms.—Great distress, slobbering, champing the jaws, escape of saliva through the nostrils, and frequent attempts at vomiting, the head being drawn toward the chest and then suddenly shot out. If the obstruction is in the neck it may easily be seen and felt.

Treatment.—Pass the hand into the pharynx and remove the obstruction if within reach. This failing, place the animal in a stall free from food and bedding, and put a bucket of water within easy reach. In the course of a few hours the obstruction is usually swallowed. It may, however, remain in the throat for a day or two. Further treatment is surgical

Diseases of the Stomach and Intestines.

412. Chronic indigestion.—A chronic inflammation of the stomach and intestines.

Causes.—Irregularity in feeding and watering, food poor in quality (spoiled or coarse), worms, old age, and improper mastication, due to bad teeth or to eating too rapidly.

Symptoms.—Appetite irregular, depraved, or diminished; constipation, usually, though there may be diarrhea. Periodic colics are frequent, the coat is rough, and the skin is tightly adherent to the body (hidebound). The animal has an unthrifty appearance and sweats and tires easily when at work. The presence of worms is recognized by their appearance in the feces, and by the presence of white patches of dried mucus around the anus.

Treatment.—Examine the mouth and correct existing faults; examine the forage and discontinue it if bad. Feed small quantities of good nutritious food (steamed oats, bran mashes, grass, etc.) at regular intervals; keep a lump of salt where the animal can reach it; give plenty of fresh drinking water, and see that the animal is regularly exercised and properly groomed.

If constipation exists, feed bran mashes or grass until the feces become soft, then give the following tonic·

	Ounces.
Gentian, powdered	3
Nux vomica, powdered	1
Bicarbonate of soda	3
Potassium nitrate	3

Mix and make into 12 powders. Give a powder twice a day.

Worms are to be removed by turpentine and raw linseed oil, as prescribed in paragraph 329, or 1 ounce of *creolin* in 1 quart of water may be given on an empty stomach. The following is also useful:

	Ounces.
Iron sulphate	1½
Gentian, powdered	3

Mix and divide into 12 powders. Give a powder morning and evening. When the last powder has been given, give 1½ pints of *raw linseed oil*.

413. Spasmodic colic (fig. 47)—Spasm of the muscular wall of the intestines.

Causes.—Sudden chilling of the body due to large drinks of cold water, or exposure to cold drafts or rains; improper feeding; indigesti-

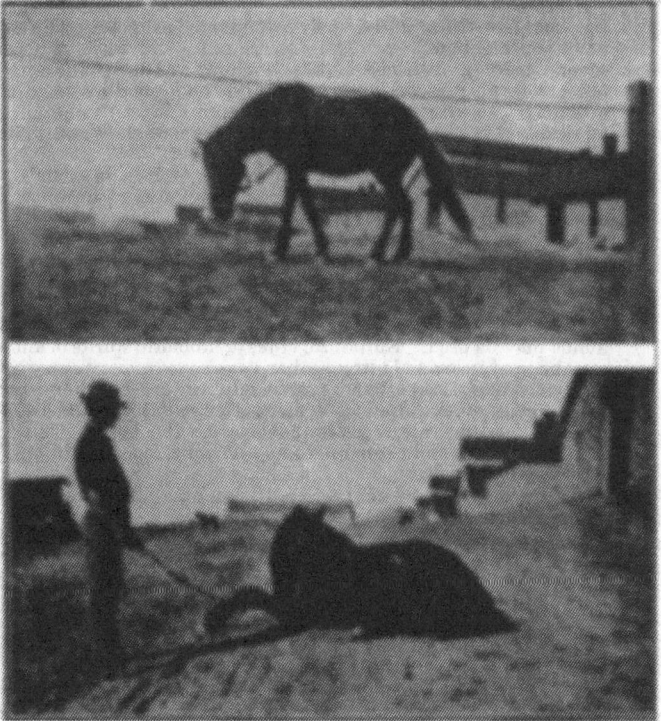

FIG. 47.—Spasmodic colic.

ble food; frozen food; and sudden changes from one variety of food to another.

Symptoms —Sudden and more or less violent attacks of pain, lasting from 5 to 10 minutes, with a tendency to recur. The animal paws, walks about, sweats profusely, rolls, and when the pain is severe, may throw himself violently down. During the attacks a few pellets of dung may be passed, and the animal may strain as if attempting to urinate. The latter symptom must not be mistaken for kidney trouble. The temperature is normal or only slightly elevated.

Treatment —Place the animal in a large, well-bedded stall, or on a soft spot of ground where there is plenty of room to roll without danger, then give the following drench:

```
Spirits nitrous ether......................ounces..   2
Cannabis indica..........................drams..   3
Water to make a pint.
```

(In the absence of cannabis indica, 1 dram fluid extract of belladonna may be used. Sulphuric ether or aromatic spirits of ammonia may be used instead of nitrous ether)

Give at one dose. If there is no relief in one-half hour, give 1½ pints *linseed oil* or 6 drams of *aloes* Give rectal injections of 5 or 6 gallons of warm water. Rub and massage the belly. The spirits of nitrous ether and cannabis indica may be repeated in one hour if necessary.

Withhold food for 12 hours after all pain has disappeared, and feed sparingly for the next day or two.

414. Flatulent colic (wind colic).—A painful affection of the stomach and bowels due to their distention with gas.

Causes.—Improper foods, such as musty or moldy oats or corn, or sour bran; green foods, as corn, clover, and alfalfa, especially when eaten wet or frosted; new hay and new oats; sudden changes of diet, and feeding animals that are overheated and exhausted. The disease is frequently observed in wind-suckers and cribbers.

Symptoms.—Bloating and swelling of the abdomen; continuous colicky pains, mild at first, but increasing in severity as the abdomen becomes more and more distended with gas. There are no periods of ease as in spasmodic colic. The animal may lie down, but for a short time only. Walking is painful, breathing is rapid and difficult, and there is great restlessness. Temperature normal or slightly elevated.

Treatment.—Put the animal in a comfortable place and drench at once with 1½ pints of *linseed oil* and two ounces of *turpentine*. If there is great pain, drench as directed in paragraph 413. Give frequent injections of 5 or 6 gallons of warm water and apply blankets wrung out in hot water to the belly.

When the above remedies are not at hand, give 6 drams of *aloes* and 4 drams of *salicylic acid* in two capsules or made up into two balls.

Another excellent remedy to be kept on hand for colics of *all* kinds is prepared as follows:

	Ounces.
Camphor gum	6
Carbolic acid	2
Glycerine	12

Mix the camphor and carbolic acid and let stand for 12 hours, then add the glycerine. Dose 1 ounce, given either in a capsule or on the tongue with a syringe. The dose may be repeated in two, four, or six hours, as indicated

When the animal has recovered, feed as directed for spasmodic colic (par. 413).

415. Obstruction colic (impaction of the intestines, stoppage of the bowels).—A painful affection of the bowels due to the accumulation of food or other material within them.

Causes.—Heavy feeding and lack of exercise; coarse, indigestible food; accumulation of sand and dirt in the bowels when horses are fed from the ground or picketed on sand (sand colic) or when watered in shallow pools or streams; insufficient water supply, and faulty mastication due to defective teeth.

Symptoms.—Constipation, dullness, and partial or complete loss of appetite. As time goes on the animal begins to show signs of restlessness and pain, such as pawing, walking round the stall, and occasionally looking around at the flank. He finally lies down, stretches himself out and remains in that position for perhaps an hour or more at a time. If relief is not given the abdomen becomes distended with gas, breathing is rapid and difficult, the pain increases in severity, and death results in from one to three or four days.

Treatment—A drench composed of *raw linseed oil* 1½ pints, and *turpentine* 2 ounces should be given at once. If pain is severe, add 4 drams *cannabis iridica* to the dose. Allow all the water the animal will drink; give rectal injections of large quantities (5 to 6 gallons) of warm water every two or three hours; rub or knead the abdominal walls, and give from five to ten minutes walking exercise every hour. If the bowels do not move within 24 hours repeat the oil and turpentine.

416. Enteritis (inflammation of the intestines).

Causes.—Sudden chilling of the body; drinking large quantities of cold water, particularly when the animal is tired and overheated; frozen or frost covered food and food that is musty or moldy; sudden changes from old to new feed; irritating medicines; blows on the abdomen, and twist or obstruction in the intestine   It sometimes follows such diseases as flatulent and spasmodic colics

Symptoms.—Intense and continuous colicky pain; temperature 103 to 106; mucous membranes of the mouth, nostrils, and eyes red and congested; the belly is tucked up and sensitive to pressure, and there is an anxious expression about the face.   The animal shows great restlessness, paws, walks about the stall, lies down carefully, rolls, and may try to balance himself on his back.   As the disease progresses, gangrene (death) of the bowels sets in after which all pain ceases and the animal stands quietly for several hours.   Toward the last he sighs, breaths hard, staggers, pitches about, falls and dies in a state of delirium.   The disease is usually fatal, the majority of cases dying in from six hours to several days.

Treatment.—Give one-half ounce *cannabis indica* in a pint of *raw* linseed oil; apply blankets wrung out in hot water to the abdomen, and give frequent rectal injections of lukewarm water.   The cannabis may be repeated in three-quarters of an hour if the pain is not relieved.   In the absence of *cannabis indica*, 2 drams *fluid extract* or *belladonna* may be used.   During convalesence feed steamed oats, bran mashes, oatmeal gruel, etc.

417. Diarrhea.—A frequent discharge of fluid or semifluid evacuations from the bowels.

Causes —Sudden changes in diet, particularly from a dry one to a moist one; musty or moldy food; large drafts of cold water when heated; worms; foreign substances as sand or dirt in the intestines and excessive use of purgatives.   Animals of a weak constitution and those of a nervous temperament often suffer without apparent cause.

Symptoms.—Frequent evacuations of soft or fluid feces.

Treatment.—Give 1½ pints *raw linseed oil*.   If there is no improvement after the action of the oil has subsided, give *tannic acid* ½ dram and 1 dram of *gum camphor*.   Repeat every four hours until the diarrhea is diminished, but not until it has become completely checked. If the feces have an offensive odor, give an ounce of *creolin* in a pint of water three times a day; or 1-ounce doses of the *camphor, carbolic acid,* and *glycerin* preparation (see par. 414) may be given three times daily If worms are known to be the cause, treat as prescribed in paragraph 412.

CHAPTER X.

DISEASES OF THE RESPIRATORY SYSTEM.

Diseases of the Nose.

418. Acute nasal catarrh (cold in the head).—An acute inflammation of the membrane lining the nasal chambers and sinuses.

Causes.—Exposure to wet and cold, particularly when tired and heated; damp, poorly ventilated stables, and sudden changes in temperature, i. e., from warm to cold.

Symptoms.—In the early stages there is sneezing or blowing and redness of the mucous membrane of the nose. Later a watery discharge appears, which soon becomes thick and of a grayish or yellowish color. The membranes of the eyes and mouth are reddened and the eyes are watery. In severe cases the disease is ushered in by a chill (shivering), elevation of temperature, and loss of appetite.

Treatment.—Place the animal in an isolated stall which is dry, well ventilated, and free from drafts. Blanket the body, hand rub the legs and bandage them loosely with flannel. Feed bran mashes, steamed oats, gruels, etc., and keep plenty of fresh water where the animal can readily reach it. Give one-half ounce *potassium nitrate* in the feed or drinking water three times daily, or *ammonium chloride* may be given instead of the potassium nitrate. The following prescription is excellent in the treatment of all catarrhal conditions.

Ammonium chloride......................ounces.. 3
Quinine sulphate ....drams... 6
Potassium nitrate.........................ounces.. 3

Mix and make into 12 powders. Give a powder three times a day.

After isolating the affected animal, thoroughly disinfect his stall, his equipment, the watering trough, and everything with which he has come in contact. This rule should be observed in all catarrhal diseases in which there is a discharge from the nose.

419. Chronic nasal catarrh (nasal gleet).—A chronic inflammation of the membrane lining the nasal chambers and sinuses.

Causes.—Chronic nasal catarrh sometimes develops from the acute. It may result from tumors in the nasal chambers, inflammation of the mucous membrane of the sinuses, or from ulceration of the teeth with filling of the sinuses with pus.   It may also accompany glanders, chronic pharyngitis, and various other diseases of the respiratory tract.

Symptoms.—The principal symptom is a persistent nasal discharge of mucus and pus, the quantity and color of which varies greatly; it may be creamy, grayish, or tinged with blood.   It is usually from one nostril only and frequently has a fetid odor.   In cases of long standing the submaxillary lymph glands are sometimes enlarged, and small ulcers which heal without leaving a scar may form in the nose.   The temperature is usually normal.

Treatment.—A careful examination of the nostrils, mouth, and teeth should be made to determine, if possible, the exact cause. If no definite cause can be found, give tonics and plenty of good food. The following prescription is useful:

> Nux vomica, powdered..................... drams .. 6
> Iron sulphate..................... ....do.... 6
> Copper sulphate.... .. ..do.... 6
> Gentian, powdered....... ....ounces.. 1½

Mix and make into 12 powders.   Give a powder three times a day.

When the disease is due to faulty teeth or to pus in the sinuses, the treatment is surgical.

420. Bleeding from the nose.

Causes —Blows about the head, injuries to the mucous membrane of the nasal cavity, and violent exertion.   It may occur during the course of such diseases as purpura hemorrhagica, influenza, nasal catarrh, glanders, and pneumonia, and is often a symptom of tumors and ulcers in the nose.

Symptoms —Bleeding from one or both nostrils, the blood escaping drop by drop or in a stream.

Treatment.—Many cases often require no treatment other than rest in a quiet place.   This failing, the head should be elevated and cold water or ice packs applied over the face, between the eyes, and over the poll and neck.

If the bleeding persists, plug the bleeding nostril with gauze, cotton, or oakum, either dry or soaked in *tincture of chloride of iron.* Wrap the plug in gauze or thin cloth and attach a string before it is pushed into the nostril, so that it can be removed after the bleeding has stopped, usually within four or five hours.   When both nostrils are bleeding, plug only one nostril at a time.   If the patient is restless, give one-half ounce *cannabis indica.*

DISEASES OF THE THROAT.

421. Laryngitis and pharyngitis (sore throat).—An inflammation of the membrane lining the larynx and pharynx.

Causes.—Chilling, due to exposure to draft, cold rains, and sudden changes of temperature, i. e , from warm to cold; infection; improper ventilation; bruises; injuries to the pharynx from foreign bodies, and irritating medicines.

Symptoms.—Difficulty in swallowing, manifested by the return through the nostrils of water and food. Diminution of appetite, cough, and stiffness of the neck. The nose is poked out, there is more or less slobbering, and pressure on the throat causes pain. There is usually a nasal discharge mixed with saliva and particles of food. The mucous membranes of the eyes, nostrils, and mouth are reddened and swollen, and breathing is often difficult and quickened. The temperature rises from 2° to 6° above normal, and there is swelling of the lymph glands of the lower jaw and throat.

Treatment —Isolate the animal in a dry, well ventilated place. Blanket warmly and bandage the legs. Feed sloppy bran mashes, grass, gruels, or steamed oats. Supply an abundance of fresh drinking water. Give one-half ounce of *ammonium chloride* or *potassium nitrate* in the drinking water morning and evening. The bucket or vessel in which the water is given should be supported in the stall at a height of 3 or 4 feet from the floor, this to enable the animal to drink without bending the neck. The lips and nostrils should be kept clean and the mouth should be washed several times a day with fresh water. In severe cases with marked heat and pain about the throat, apply cold compresses. In mild cases *ammonia liniment* may be used. If the temperature is high, give frequent rectal injections of 2 or 3 gallons of cold water. Do not drench or give balls.

The following is a suitable prescription:

Fluid extract belladonna	dram	½
Pine tar	do	1
Glycerine	ounce	½

This makes one dose. Mix and smear on the back of the tongue and back teeth with a thin stick; give morning and evening until relief is afforded.

106233°—17——9

DISEASES OF THE LUNGS.

422. Pneumonia.—An inflammation of lung structure affecting one or both lungs.

Causes.—Over exertion; badly ventilated stables; exposure to cold, especially when heated; infection, and carelessness in drenching.

Symptoms.—A severe chill, with a temperature varying from 103° to 107°. Then follows redness of the visible mucous membranes; rapid, difficult breathing, and a full rapid pulse (from 50 to 80 per minute). The nostrils are dilated and the expired air is quite warm. The animal is usually constipated at first, and the urine is scanty and high-colored. The legs and ears are cold and there is great weakness. The patient may remain constantly standing with the elbows turned out and the head drooping, or it may lie down for a short time only. There is frequently a reddish discharge from the nose and there may or may not be a cough

Treatment.—Isolate the animal in a clean, dry place free from drafts, but abundantly supplied with fresh air. Clothe the body according to the season; rub the legs well and bandage with flannel. Remove the bandages twice daily, rub the legs well, and reapply. Groom as directed in paragraph 214. Feed easily digested food (bran mashes, grass, good hay, and steamed oats), and keep a supply of fresh water within reach at all times. Give one-ounce *nitrate of potassium* in the drinking water morning and evening. If the temperature reaches 105° or more, give rectal injections of cold water three or four times a day. For great weakness, give *nitrous ether* (2 ounces) in the drinking water three times daily. When the temperature begins to subside, tonics are indicated. Do not put the animal to work for at least a month after all symptoms have disappeared.

423. Heaves (broken wind).—A chronic, nonfebrile disease of the lungs.

Causes.—Violent and prolonged exertion; working the animal when his stomach and intestines are distended with food, or when he is suffering or convalescing from diseases of the respiratory organs; or, the habitual feeding of coarse, bulky, dusty, and indigestible food, and foods that are damaged by mold, rust, or decay.

Symptoms.—A hurried, wheezy, laborious breathing; a double lifting of the flanks with each expiration; a short, weak, dry cough;

a thin, watery, intermittent nasal discharge, and frequent expulsions of large quantities of gas from the rectum.

The symptoms are aggravated by damp, muggy weather, by exercise, and by dusty, coarse foods and overfeeding.

Treatment.—The disease is incurable and treatment gives only relief.

See that the forage is of the best; water before feeding; dampen the food, and feed often and in small amounts. Feed more grain and less hay, and give bran mashes, grass, or other laxative foods at least three times a week. Allow the animal to rest for one hour after feeding, and work slowly.

CHAPTER XI.

DISEASES OF THE UROGENITAL SYSTEM.

Diseases of the Kidneys.

424. Acute inflammation of the kidneys (nephritis).—A rare disease of the horse.

Causes.—Obstruction to the ureters; musty food; certain poisonous plants; exposure to cold; the internal administration of large or continued doses of turpentine; and the application of cantharides blisters over large areas of the body. Most cases are secondary to infectious diseases.

Symptoms.—Fever; hard and frequent pulse, with complete or partial suppression of urine, the latter being sometimes the color of blood. The animal stands with arched back and legs spread apart; it dislikes to move, and if forced to do so the hind legs are dragged; there is great uneasiness; and pressure on the loins causes pain.

Treatment.—Remove the cause and give absolute rest. Avoid all irritating drugs, and provide a diet of grass, bran mashes, or other easily digested foods. Corn, oats, and grain of all kinds must be withheld. In case of marked decrease in the quantity of urine, plenty of pure, fresh drinking water must be provided. Give *linseed oil* 1½ pints, and apply blankets wrung out in hot water to the loins. Keep the patient in a warm stall, rub the body vigorously, blanket well and bandage the legs. Give *potassium nitrate* one-half ounce twice daily in the drinking water.

425. Diabetes insipidus (excessive urination).—A condition characterized by great thirst, excessive urination, marked debility and rapid loss of flesh.

Causes.—Moldy food, especially oats; certain poisonous plants, and the long continued administration of diuretics, as turpentine and the nitrate of potassium.

Symptoms.—Frequent passages of large quantities of clear, water-like urine, the total amounting to from 10 to 15 gallons in 24 hours; great thirst, the animal drinking as much as 20 or 25 gallons of water in a day.

Treatment.—Remove the cause and give good, clean, and nutritious food. If a change of diet is impossible, the forage at hand may be

130

rendered less harmful by spreading it out and exposing it to the sun and air. Feed grass whenever obtainable. Give *iodine crystals* in 1-dram doses three times a day in capsule or ball, and reduce the dose as the thirst is lessened and the amount of urine diminished.

Diseases of the Bladder.

426. Retention of the urine.—Inability to urinate.

Causes.—Hard, continuous work without an opportunity to urinate; exposure to cold rains; standing in drafts of cold air when hot and tired; the presence of stones or tumors in the bladder or urethra, and poisonous plants in the hay. It also frequently occurs in a temporary form as a complication of colic. Some horses refuse to urinate outside of their own stable, or where the floor or earth is hard causing the urine to splash against their legs. A collection of dirt about the end of the penis may also cause it.

Symptoms.—Frequent and painful attempts to urinate, the urine often being passed drop by drop only. By passing the hand into the rectum the enlarged bladder may be felt.

Treatment.—Standing the animal on the grass or in a well-bedded stall often results in successful attempts to urinate. This failing, pass the hand into the rectum and apply firm but gentle pressure to the base of the bladder. If neither of these methods is successful, the catheter must be used or the bladder may burst. Warm rectal injections and 3-dram doses *cannabis indica* often gives relief. When retention is due to a collection of dirt in the end of the penis, a thorough washing of the part may be all that is required.

Diseases of the Sheath and Penis.

427. Screw worms (maggots) in the sheath and penis.— Screw worms are the immature forms of several species of flies. During hot weather and in tropical climates these flies frequently deposit their eggs just inside the mouth of the sheath, usually in its upper portion, or on the end of the penis. In a few hours the eggs hatch and large numbers of maggots appear which immediately lacerate the skin and burrow into the tissues where they produce destruction and injury, even to perforations of the abdominal wall.

Symptoms.—A thin bloody serum dripping from the mouth of the sheath, the latter being often more or less swollen. Just inside of the sheath, beneath the abdominal wall, may be found a small,

irregular wound discharging a thin bloody fluid.   Within this wound
the maggots may be seen.   In case no abrasions are found within the
sheath, the penis should be withdrawn and carefully examined, pay-
ing particular attention to the two small pockets at the sides of the
mouth of the urethra.

Treatment —With forceps pick out all the worms that are visible,
and wipe out the cavity with a swab of cotton that has been saturated
in a solution of *carbolic acid* 1 part to 5 parts of water.   Creolin full
strength may be used in the same way, or the wound may be packed
with *calomel*.   *Turpentine* 1 part, *olive oil* 3 parts is also useful.
After the worms are killed, the wound should be treated with ordinary antiseptics.

CHAPTER XII.

DISEASES OF THE CIRCULATORY AND LYMPHATIC SYSTEM.

DISEASES OF THE CIRCULATORY SYSTEM.

428. Edema of the legs (stocking, dropsy of the legs, filled legs).—A chronic condition of the legs in which there is more or less swelling.

Causes.—Debility, heavy feeding, and lack of exercise.

Symptoms.—Moderate, nonpainful swelling of one or both hind legs which disappears more or less by exercise and returns after the animal has stood in the stable for some time. The swelling may sometimes extend to the sheath and belly. The fore legs are rarely affected.

Treatment.—Laxative diet. Regular exercise. Hand rub and bandage the legs immediately after the animal returns from work. Tonics.

DISEASES OF THE LYMPHATIC SYSTEM.

429. Acute lymphangitis (fig 48) —An acute inflammation of the lymphatics of one or more limbs, usually a hind one, seldom a fore one.

Causes.—High feeding and irregular exercise. The disease seldom occurs in animals that are regularly worked. It is usually seen in those that, in the midst of hard work, are kept idle in the stable for two or three days on the same ration they had while working.

Symptoms.—Loss of appetite, great thirst, shivering, labored breathing, rapid pulse, and high temperature (104°–106°). The animal dislikes to move and if forced to do so, it shows great lameness in one hind limb, which at each step is carried outward well away from the opposite leg. The inside of the thigh of the affected limb is swollen, hot, and exceedingly painful to the touch. If not relieved, the swelling gradually increases until the limb becomes two or three times its natural thickness. There is usually constipation, and the urine is scanty and high-colored.

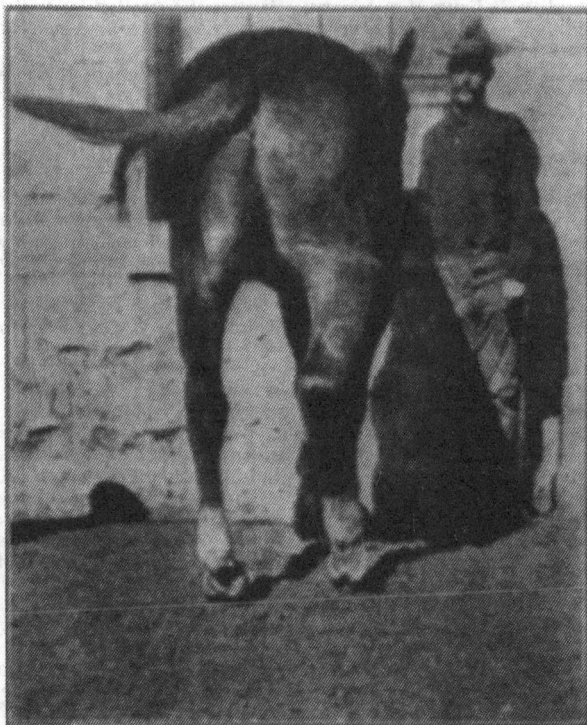

FIG. 48.—Acute lymphangitis.

Treatment.—Give 1½ pints of *linseed oil* at once Add 1 ounce of *potassium nitrate* to the drinking water three times a day. Repeat the oil in 24 hours if necessary. Shower the swollen leg with cold water for 20 minutes three or four times a day and follow each shower with a white lotion (half strength) bath or pack. When the pain has diminished, give slow walking exercise followed immediately by warm baths and gentle hand rubbing. Allow plenty of drinking water and feed grass, bran mashes, and other laxative foods.

DISEASES OF THE BLOOD AND BLOOD-PRODUCING ORGANS.

430. Azoturia.—An acute disease of horses and mules characterized by *coffee-colored urine* and severe *disturbances in the movement of the hind limbs.* The disease occurs most frequently in highly-fed horses in good muscular condition and accustomed to regular work. It usually follows a rest of two or three days and appears when the animal is again put to work. The condition is rare in poorly nourished horses and in horses that are regularly worked and properly fed.

Causes.—Feeding full rations during a short period (two or three days) of rest in the stable, the horse being used to regular work.

Symptoms.—The attack usually comes on suddenly and within 20 minutes after leaving the stable. Without any visible cause the animal, which has been playful and full of life, suddenly becomes excited, knuckles in one or both hind fetlocks, and acts as if he had been badly injured about the loins, croup, and thighs. The muscles of these regions soon become swollen and hard; they tremble and contract violently, but are not sensitive to pressure. The hind legs are stiff and usually advanced, and, in attempting to put weight on them, the hind quarters often drop until the hocks touch the ground. The breathing is rapid, perspiration is profuse, and the animal is in great agony. There is usually constipation. The urine is *coffee-colored* and often retained in the bladder. The muscles of the fore limbs and shoulders are sometimes involved, but not often. Sometimes the symptoms are mild, but if urged on, the animal falls to the ground and struggles until it dies in a few days or a week. Mild cases which are stopped before they *go down* usually recover.

Treatment.—Stop the animal immediately the first symptoms are observed. To move him at once to the nearest stable is unwise. Immediate and absolute rest is essential to recovery. Even the hauling of the patient to the stable should be forbidden, as the struggling and excitement produced by the procedure will surely convert even a mild case into a hopeless one.

Remove the saddle or harness at once; keep the animal standing, if possible; if not, provide a good bed. Cover the body with two or three blankets and bandage the legs. Heat some oats or common salt, which place in a sack and spread over the loins; or, weather permitting, saturate blankets in warm water and apply in the same way. Give 2 ounces *spirits nitrous ether* and 4 drams *cannabis indica*, and in one-half hour give a cathartic. If there is retention of the urine, empty the bladder three times a day by passing the hand into the rectum and applying firm pressure to the bladder.

If the patient is down, give a good bed and turn animal over every two or three hours. Provide plenty of fresh drinking water and feed bran mashes, grass, and hay. The animal should not be worked for four to six weeks after all symptoms have disappeared.

Prevention.—Exercise all animals daily. When this is impossible, reduce the grain ration one-half and feed bran mashes or grass.

CHAPTER XIII.

DISEASES OF THE NERVOUS SYSTEM.

431. Congestion of the brain.—An accumulation of blood in the vessels of the brain.

Causes.—Diseases of the heart, over exertion, excitement, extreme heat, pressure on the jugular veins (a tight collar), or compression of the lungs due to bloating of the stomach or intestines.

Symptoms —In mild cases the animal is restless and excited, the eyes are bright and the pupils dilated. The cranium feels abnormally hot and the mucous membranes of the head are injected.

Other cases are characterized by depression. The animal may stop very suddenly and shake his head or stand quietly braced on his legs, then stagger, make a plunge, and fall   The eyes are staring, the breathing is hurried and snoring, and the nostrils are widely dilated. This may be followed by coma (stupor), violent convulsive movements, and death. Generally, however, the animal gains relief in a short time, but may remain weak and giddy for several days

Treatment —Prompt removal of too tight a collar or other mechanical obstruction to the circulation will give immediate relief. If the animal is partially or totally unconscious, apply cold water or ice packs to the head. When able to swallow, give 1½ to 2 pints of *raw linseed oil*. Put the animal in a quiet, well-ventilated stall and feed a laxative diet. If the disease is caused by bloating, treat as directed in paragraph 414.

432. Concussion of the brain.—A bruising of the brain, the result of injury to any part of the head.

Causes.—Concussion of the brain is generally caused by an animal falling over backward and striking his poll, or by kicks, blows, or collisions.

Symptoms.—Giddiness, stupor, unconsciousness, or loss of muscular power, appearing as a rule immediately after the animal has been injured. In other cases, some minutes elapse before their appearance. The animal may recover quickly or not for hours. Death may occur on the spot or after a few days.

137

Treatment.—In mild cases the animal quickly regains its feet and no treatment is required. Keep the patient quiet for a few days and give a laxative diet. In more severe cases, where there is more or less loss of consciousness, cold in the form of water or ice should be applied to the head. It may be necessary to continue these applications for hours. If the animal is down, the head should be raised several inches from the ground and the patient made as comfortable as possible. If, after an hour of this treatment the animal is able to swallow, a stimulant, such as *aromatic spirits of ammonia* or *spirits of nitrous ether*, should be given and repeated in an hour. When the animal regains consciousness it should be assisted to rise, and then thoroughly hand-rubbed all over.

The after treatment consists in keeping the animal quiet, giving laxative food, and adding one-half ounce of *potassium nitrate* to the drinking water twice a day.

If there is a wound on the head it must be treated as directed under treatment of wounds.

433. Sunstroke and heatstroke.—Disturbances of the nervous system due to exposure to heat.

Causes.—Exposure to the direct rays of the sun or to extreme heat from any source.

Symptoms—In the early stages the animal appears dull and depressed. If at work it requires urging. The gait is uncertain and stumbling, breathing is difficult and snoring, and the expression of the face is anxious. The nostrils are dilated and the mucous membrane lining the nasal cavities is at first red and congested, but later becomes pale and often bluish. The temperature may be as high as 108° or over. Later on there is violent trembling and the animal may fall and die in convulsions, or it may lie unconscious for several hours or days, finally recovering or dying.

Treatment.—If possible, the animal should be placed in a cool, shady spot or in water, and cold water poured over the body, the head and the neck. If practicable, ice packs should be applied to the head. Give rectal injections of cold water and rub the body vigorously and often.

When the animal is able to swallow, a good stimulant, such as *aromatic spirits of ammonia* or *spirits of nitrous ether* in 2-ounce doses, well diluted, should be given and repeated in an hour. In the cool of the evening or early morning the animal may be moved, if necessary, but should be kept in a cool place during the heat of the day until recovery is perfect.

434. Spasm of the diaphragm (thumps).—A spasmodic contraction of the muscles of the diaphragm.

Causes.—Diseases of the digestive organs and over exertion.

Symptoms.—A convulsive jerking of the body, most marked in the left flank, and frequently accompanied by a loud thumping noise. Trembling, restlessness, distress, and yawning are seen in some cases.

Treatment.—Place the animal in a quiet place where there is plenty of fresh air, but free from drafts. Give stimulants and antispasmodics such as *aromatic spirits of ammonia*, 1½ ounces, and *cannabis indica*, 2 to 4 drams in a pint of water. Repeat in one hour if necessary. When the disease is caused by digestive disturbances, treat as prescribed in chapter on diseases of the digestive system.

CHAPTER XIV.

DISEASES OF THE EYE.

435. Conjunctivitis.—An inflammation of the conjunctiva.

Causes.—Foreign bodies in the eye such as dust, insects, chaff, sand, hair, etc., and injuries from whips, branches, and stubbles. Also irritating gases, glare of the sun, microbes, and infectious diseases.

Symptoms.—The discharge of tears, redness of the conjunctiva, and the closure more or less complete of the eyelids are the first and most marked symptoms. Later the lids become swollen and completely closed, or the haw partially covers the cornea. The discharge becomes thicker and mats the eyelashes together, or holds the eyelids closed. Unless the cornea has been directly injured it usually remains clear. Mild cases usually recover in a week or 10 days.

Treatment.—The first step is to remove the cause. Foreign bodies may be removed by washing out the eye with clean, warm water, or by the careful use of a tightly rolled swab of cotton or gauze. This failing, the forceps may be used. Place the animal in the shade or in a dark stall and cover the eye with a clean cloth on the inside of which a piece of absorbent cotton covered with gauze has been sewed. Keep the cotton wet with a saturated solution of *boric acid*. Twice a day a few drops of the following solution should be placed in the eye:

Zinc sulphate.............................grains..	20
Boric acid................................dram..	1
Water....................................ounces..	4

Mix. Use as above directed.

436. Acute keratitis.—An inflammation of the cornea.

Causes.—Wounds of the cornea by foreign bodies, particles of glass, blows of whips, chaff, etc.

Symptoms.—The eye is extremely sensitive, and usually kept closed. There is a profuse flow of tears, and a disposition to resist opening of the lids. When exposed the cornea is seen to be more or less clouded and perhaps reddened by the formation of blood

140

vessels proceeding from its sclerotic margin. The cloudiness increases to a deep white opacity. In severe cases the cornea may become of a bright pink color, and abscesses or ulcers may form.

Treatment.—Any foreign body adhering to the cornea must be removed and the eye washed out with a saturated solution of *boric acid.* The eye is then covered as directed in conjunctivitis and treated in the same way. The opacity (cloudiness) remaining after the inflammation has subsided may be removed by the application of a few drops of the following solution:

> Silver nitrate...........................grains.. 2
> Water....................................ounce.. 1

Mix. Place a few drops in the eye once a day.

437. Recurrent ophthalmia (periodic ophthalmia).—An inflammatory condition of the interior of the eye, intimately related to certain constitutions, soils, climates, and systems of management, showing a strong tendency to recur again and again and usually ending in blindness from cataract or other destructive lesions.

Causes.—A wet, impervious, swampy, or undrained soil. Any debilitating disease, overwork, insufficient or indigestible food, and local irritants, such as blows on the eye, dust, and other foreign bodies. Also infection.

Symptoms.—In some cases there is high fever, in others this may be absent. The attack is sudden, the eyelids are closed, and the tears run down the face. The conjunctiva is red and congested, and the outer border of the cornea is clouded. In a few days the cloudiness extends over the entire cornea, and a grayish yellow sediment frequently appears in the anterior chamber just back of the cornea. Attacks last from 10 to 15 days, and reappear in from 30 to 60 days. From five to seven attacks usually result in blindness, and then the other eye is likely to suffer a similar attack until both are ruined.

Treatment.—Treat as for conjunctivitis In addition provide good healthful surroundings and give a good tonic, as follows:

	Ounces
Iron sulphate....................................	1
Gentian, powdered..............................	1½
Nux vomica.....................................	1½

Mix and make 12 powders. Give a powder twice a day in feed.

438. Cataract.—Opacity of the lens or of its capsule.

Causes.—Usually results from repeated attack or recurrent ophthalmia.

Symptoms.—Blindness, and opacity or cloudiness of the lens. The lens turns white and is no longer transparent as in the healthy eye.

Treatment.—No treatment will restore the eye to its normal condition.

439. Wounds of the eyelids.

Causes.—Kicks, and tears by nails or other sharp objects.

Treatment.—Clean the part thoroughly, removing all dried blood, pus, hair, and dirt, and draw the edges of the wound together with a fine needle and a piece of silk thread, being careful not to injure the eye. When the stitches are all in, touch the edges of the wound with *tincture of iodine* and dust with *boric acid* or *iodoform.* Care must be taken not to let the iodine enter the eye. When the parts are badly swollen, apply a pad of cotton and gauze and keep it saturated as prescribed for conjunctivitis (par. 435). Dress the wound daily as directed in paragraphs 355 and 359. The animal must be cross tied or in some way prevented from injuring the wound.

CHAPTER XV.

DISEASES OF THE SKIN.

440. Eczema.—An acute or chronic inflammatory disease of the skin characterized by lesions of many forms and the presence of more or less itching. In the Philippines it often assumes an aggravated form and is improperly called "Dhobie itch"

Causes.—External irritants, as the accumulation and decomposition of dirt among the hairs; constant dampness of the skin from rain, washing or sweating, causing a softening of its outer layers and favoring the growth of fungi and other vegetable parasites, and exposure to the hot rays of the sun, especially when the skin is damp It may appear under the saddle, under the harness, or at any point where chafing and sweating occur, and it may accompany digestive disturbances and other debilitating diseases.

Symptoms—The skin is reddened, pimpled, blistered, and sometimes cracked. The blisters break, their fluid escapes, dries and forms scabs and crusts around the roots of the hairs which later fall out. These lesions may be limited to certain regions or they may cover the whole surface of the body.

Treatment.—When due to indigestion, give 1½-ounce doses of *sodium bicarbonate* twice a day in the drinking water.

Clip the hair from the diseased parts. When scabs and crusts are formed, soften them for 24 hours with *creolin* ½ ounce and *olive oil* 10 ounces. Wash off with warm water, soap and brush; then apply *creolin* 1 ounce and *olive oil* 10 ounces once a day until the skin is healthy.

Regulate the diet and give tonics Do not use the patients grooming outfit, blanket, or bridle on other animals until they have been disinfected.

441. Scratches (cracked heels).—An acute inflammation of the skin of the legs, usually that of the posterior part of the pastern.

Causes.—Close, dirty stables; standing in dung, urine, and slush; washing and insufficiently drying the legs, and allowing horses with wet legs to stand in a draft.

White legs are said to suffer more than others This is not because they are white, but because it is the white leg that gets the most washing.

Symptoms.—The skin is hot, painful, and more or less swollen. It may crack, and on it little blisters may form, followed by an oily fetid exudate. There is usually lameness.

Treatment —Rest; bran mashes; grass, etc ; *potassium nitrate*, 2 drams in drinking water morning and evening.

Cleanse the diseased parts with castile soap and water, dry, and apply a *white lotion* pack twice daily; or, the following preparation may be used:

	Ounce.
Tincture iodine	1
Tincture chloride of iron	1
Glycerine	1

Mix. Apply twice a day.

When the parts become dry, hard, and scabby, *oxide of zinc ointment* may be applied once or twice daily. When the parts are moist or oily, dry dressings, such as *oxide of zinc, boric acid*, or *iodoform*, either powdered on loosely or held in place by a piece of cotton and a bandage, may be used.

442. Grease (fig. 49).—A chronic inflammation of the skin of the back part of the pastern and fetlock.

Causes.—The disease usually results from a neglected case of scratches. (See Causes, par. 441.)

Symptoms.—Skin red, swollen, painful and hot, and later covered with blisters which break and discharge a thin, yellowish fluid. The hairs may be matted together or they may fall out. In the course of a few days the liquid from the blisters decomposes, resulting in the formation of a dirty, doughy, stinking deposit. If not properly treated, wartlike growths, varying in size from that of a pea to a grape may be formed. This is called the *grapy* stage, and the growths themselves are called *grapes*.

The affected leg is more or less swollen, and lameness is usually well marked.

Treatment.—In the first stages the treatment is the same as for scratches. (See par. 441.) When grapes appear they must be nipped off with the scissors and their bases burnt with *copper sulphate* or *lanar caustic*, after which the treatment is the same as for resh wounds.

443. Urticaria (nettlerash).—A disease characterized by the sudden appearance of roundish shallow elevations on the skin.

Causes.—Sudden changes of weather; unwholesome food; sudden changes of food; irritating substances to the skin, such as turpentine,

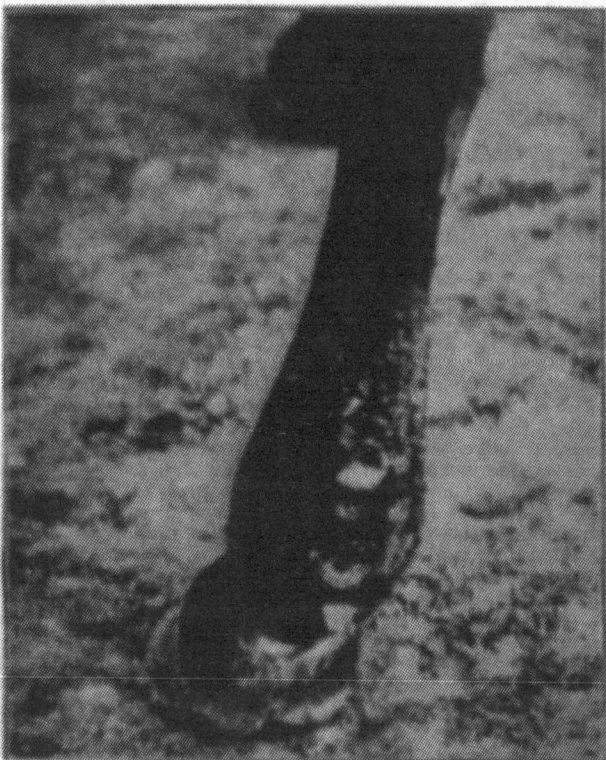

FIG. 49.—Grease.

phenol, and the secretions of ants, flies, and other insects. It may also occur as a complication of indigestion, and in the course of infectious diseases, such as strangles and influenza.

Symptoms.—Suddenly appearing roundish or oblong lumps or swellings, varying in size from that of a pea to that of a walnut, hard, flat, or half round, scattered about here and there on the skin. These swellings may develop in 5 to 30 minutes and disappear in one to two hours to two days. In some cases the swellings may occur about the nostrils, causing them to become so thickened as to interfere with breathing.

Treatment.—Give 1½ pints *linseed oil,* followed by 1-ounce doses *sodium bicarbonate* in the drinking water morning and evening for three days. If suffocation threatens, bathe the nostrils with cold water. Feed bran mashes, grass, etc., for two or three days after the symptoms disappear.

444. Stings of bees, wasps, and hornets.

Treatment.—Bathe the injured parts with *white lotion;* or a solution of *carbolic acid,* one-half ounce to a quart of water; or *potassium permanganate,* one-half teaspoonful to a pint of water; or *sodium bicarbonate,* a tablespoonful to water 1 pint. Pure, cold water may also be used.

445. Snake bites.

Symptoms.—Two or four small punctured wounds, the nature and number of which vary according to the species of the snake making them, that of the rattler showing two small, deep punctures, usually one immediately above the other. Around the bite large, doughy swellings appear, black blood may ooze from the wound, and there are pronounced symptoms of dizziness, weakness, and prostration.

Treatment.—If the bite is on a limb, tie a bandage around the leg above the wound, and draw it tight. The wound is then freely laid open with a knife and burnt with a pointed hot iron; or packed with crystals of *potassium permanganate* or *lunar caustic.* Other valuable remedies are such as *tincture of iodine* and *tincture of chloride of iron,* either of which may be injected deeply into the wound.

Internally, give *aromatic spirits of ammonia, spirits of nitrous ether, alcohol,* or *whisky* in doses of from 1 to 3 ounces.

PARASITIC DISEASES OF THE SKIN.

446. Lice.—The presence of lice is often an indication of insuffi
cient grooming and bad stable management.

Symptoms —Intense itching; loss of hair; sometimes eruptions on
the skin. A careful examination will reveal the parasites (lice).

Treatment.—Isolate the patient Wash the entire body with a
solution of *creolin* (2 ounces) and water (3 quarts). Repeat the
washings every six days until three applications have been made.
When circumstances permit, the animal should be clipped before
treatment is begun   Burn the hair.

Disinfect stall, equipment, blankets, and grooming utensils.

Tobacco tea, made by boiling 6 ounces tobacco stems for twenty
minutes in 1 gallon of water, is an excellent preparation for the
destruction of lice. With it, however, only one-half of the body
should be washed at a time, otherwise the animal may suffer from
nicotine poisoning   Twenty-four hours should elapse between the
washings.

447. Mange (scabies).—A contagious disease of the skin. May
be transmitted to man.

Causes —A very small animal parasite, the mange mite, of which
there are three varieties:

(a) The burrowing mite, which bores itself into the skin   It is
usually found about the head and neck, but occasionally also on
other parts of the body

(b) The sucking mite, which gets its nourishment by sucking the
juices from the skin   Found at the roots of the mane and tail

(c) The scale-eating mite, found on the extremities.

Symptoms —Violent, unceasing, intolerable itching of the affected
parts, the patient rubbing, scratching, and biting continuously.
The hair falls out and the skin becomes thickened, wrinkled, and
covered with scabs; or, it may become torn and raw by the never-
ending rubbing and scratching.

Treatment —This must be prompt and energetic. Isolate the
animal, clip the coat and burn the hair. Wash the diseased parts and
soften the scabs with warm water, soap, and scrubbing brush, dry,
and wash daily with *creolin*, 4½ ounces to water, 3 quarts; or apply
creolin and *oil* (1–20) twice a day and wash thoroughly every other
day with warm water and soap   Continue the treatment until the
parts are healed.   Tobacco tea, made as directed in paragraph 446 is
also a useful remedy in the treatment of mange.

Disinfect stable, troughs, picket lines, fences, equipments, blankets, grooming utensils, clothing of attendants, etc.

448. Ringworm (herpes).—A contagious disease of the skin characterized by falling out of the hair in circular isolated patches.

Causes.—A vegetable parasite.

Symptoms.—Falling out of the hair in circular patches about the size of a 25-cent piece, after which there remains an elevated, scaly eruption. The parts usually affected are the head, neck, shoulders, back, flank, croup, and sometimes the belly. Itching is not marked.

Treatment.—Isolate the patient. Cut away the hair from the diseased area; soften the scaly eruptions with a mixture of *creolin* (one-half ounce) and *olive oil* (10 ounces) which leave on for two days, then wash well with warm water and soap, and remove the soft scabs. Follow this with daily applications of *tincture of iodine*. Should the eruptions be numerous, *creolin* baths may be used. From two to three months are often required to bring about the cure.

Disinfect stall, equipment, and grooming utensils.

449. Ticks.—Ticks are small animal parasites which live on bushes and attach themselves to the skin of animals only for the purpose of sucking their blood. When filled they drop off and fall to the ground.

Treatment.—They are easily destroyed by the application of oil or grease which kills them by stopping up their breathing pores. If pulled off by the hand a part of the body sometimes breaks off and remains in the skin, often causing sores and abscesses.

450. Warbles (grubs).—Tumors on the backs of horses produced by the undeveloped form of the warble or gadfly. Common in the Southwestern States.

Symptoms.—The parasite lives under the skin of the back, where it forms an abscess about the size of a hazelnut or larger, and sucks nourishment from the surrounding tissues.

Treatment.—Make a very small opening in the abscess and squeeze out the parasite with the fingers. Treat the remaining wound with an antiseptic.

CHAPTER XVI.

DISEASES OF THE FOOT.

451. Acute laminitis (founder).—An acute inflammation of the laminar corium and its adjoining structures. It usually affects the fore feet, sometimes the hind ones in addition, but seldom the hind ones alone.

Causes—Long-continued fast work on hard roads; prolonged standing in the stable, on board ship, or on railroad cars; sudden chilling of the body, such as may arise from standing in a draft or from drinking large quantities of cold water, particularly when the animal is heated or exhausted; overfeeding; improper foods, especially foods that are musty or mouldy, and sudden changes in diet, as from old to new forage. It may also occur as a complication of colic, influenza, pneumonia, and may follow the excessive use of severe purgatives.

Symptoms.—Sudden and intense lameness. When the fore feet are affected they are planted far in advance of the body, and the hind ones are placed well forward under the belly. The affected feet are hot and painful and there is increased pulsation in the digital arteries. If forced to move, the feet are raised laboriously, the animal groans with pain, and sweat may break out over the body. In some instances the animal may lie down on his side with legs stretched out, for hours at a time; in other cases he stands continuously.

The pulse is strong and full and often increased to 80 or 90 a minute; there is muscular trembling; the respirations are short and rapid, and the temperature may rise to 105° or over.

In less severe cases, the symptoms are less marked. The animal moves stiffly, taking short, rapid steps with the fore feet, the hind ones being thrust forward to take the greater share of the weight.

Treatment.—Give 1½ pints *linseed oil* as a drench, and add 2 to 4 ounces of *potassium nitrate* to the drinking water three times a day for one or two days. If there is great pain, give 2 to 4 drams *cannabis indica* and repeat if necessary. Remove the shoes and stand the animal in a stream or a pond for five or six hours at a time each day, or apply cold packs (cracked ice, if obtainable) to the feet and legs as high as the knees and keep them wet. *Stop all grain and feed bran*

149

mashes, grass, or *hay* When the animal is not standing in water, place him in a well-bedded stall to encourage him to lie down and rest his feet, or he may be placed in slings.

If after two or three days of this treatment no improvement is observed, change to hot baths or packs, being sure that they extend as high as the knees.

As soon as the pain has diminished moderate exercise may be given and gradually increased until lameness has disappeared. If there is no improvement after five or six days of such exercise, apply a cantharides blister to the coronet and repeat in two weeks if necessary.

452. Bruises of the sole and frog.

Causes.—Stepping on stones or other hard objects.

Symptoms.—Sudden and more or less severe lameness In many cases the toe only is placed on the ground The foot is hot, there is marked throbbing in the digital arteries, and the use of the tester causes great pain.

Treatment.—Stand the animal in cold water or apply cold poultices to the foot. If, after two or three days of this treatment the foot is still hot and painful, change to poultices of hot flaxseed meal. If pus forms, remove the underrun horn and treat as directed for suppurating corns, paragraph 454.

453. Canker.—A chronic disease of the corium of the frog and sole.

Causes.—Filth and moisture. It often results from a neglected case of thrush and from injuries which expose the soft structures of the sole and frog

Symptoms.—The frog becomes large and spongy and the diseased area is covered with a half-dried, cheesy material, the odor of which is disgusting. The disease may spread until the entire frog, bars, sole, and even the wall may become involved, all having a spongy appearance and bleeding freely. Lameness is usually absent.

Treatment.—Pare the foot down carefully, remove all underrun horn, and clean the exposed parts with creolin, 1 ounce in 20 ounces of water. The soft spongy material must then be removed with the scissors. Profuse bleeding usually follows, and a pressure dressing of cotton and oakum must be applied to check it. This dressing is left in place for two or three hours, after which it must be removed and the foot wiped dry with cotton. The diseased area is then thoroughly powdered over with the three sulphates and a pressure dressing applied. Repeat this dressing daily until a new growth of horn is formed. The horse may now be shod. Pack the foot with oakum and tar and cover with a leather sole, which is held in place by the shoe.

Should it be desirable to change the dressing on the shod foot, a more convenient appliance to keep them in place is made in the following manner: Cut a piece of zinc to cover about two-thirds of the sole and frog, the outer edge of the piece fitting under the shoe; cut another piece to cover the remaining third and wide enough to lap over the first piece, the lap to run parallel with the cleft of the frog; then cut a strip about one inch wide to act as a keeper; the ends of this strip are passed under the shoe, the strip passing across the foot from quarter to quarter.

Other recommendable remedies in the treatment of canker are as follows:

A.

Formalin..................................ounces.. ⅞
Alcohol..................................do.... 9½

Apply once daily until parts become hard.

B.

Bichloride of mercury......................drams.. 2
50 per cent alcohol......................ounces.. 5

Apply gently with a soft cotton swab. When dry apply a pressure dressing.

454. Corns.—A corn is a bruise to the sensitive sole between the wall and the bar. Corns occur usually in the fore feet, where they are found more often in the inner than in the outer heel. They are seldom found in the hind feet.

Corns may be *dry* or *suppurating*.

A *dry* corn is one in which the injury is but slight, and where nothing but the staining of the horn with blood remains to indicate that an injury has existed.

A *suppurating* corn is one in which pus has formed.

Causes.—Fast work on hard roads. Improper shoeing, such as lowering one quarter more than the other; leaving the toe too long; lowering the wall too much and allowing the sole to rest on the shoe; shoeing with shoes that are too short; fitting the shoes too close at the heels, and allowing the shoes to remain on so long that the wall overgrows the heels of the shoe and causes the shoe to press on the sole.

Symptoms.—Lameness may or may not be present. When present, there is heat and tenderness in the injured quarter. Upon removal of the superficial layers of the sole at the seat of the injury, the deeper layers will be seen to be of a reddish or purplish color. Should suppuration threaten, lameness becomes well marked, the foot is quite hot, and the use of the tester causes great pain. If not relieved, the pus may break through the tissues immediately above the horn, usually at the bulb of the heel.

Treatment.—Level the foot and correct any faults that may be detected. Trim away the bearing surface of the sole and wall in such a manner that the shoe can not cause pressure upon the diseased parts, and reshoe. If the foot is hot and painful, apply cold poultices or stand the patient in cold water until the inflammation subsides. This failing, apply warm poultices until the horn softens and pus appears; then open well at the bottom; remove all horn that is underrun by pus; cleanse the parts thoroughly; apply tincture of iodine; bandage carefully, and place the patient in a clean dry stall. Dress the foot daily until lameness and suppuration cease, then plug the corn with tar and oakum, and shoe with a bar shoe.

455. Cracks in the wall of the hoof.—Most frequently found on the inner side of the front hoofs; on the hind hoofs, usually at the toe. According to location they are classified as *toe cracks* and *quarter cracks*. Cracks which affect only the upper border of the hoof are called *coronary cracks;* those affecting the lower border of the hoof are called *low cracks;* while those extending from one border to the other are called *complete cracks*.

Causes.—Weak quarters; excessive dryness of the hoof; lack of frog pressure; contracted heels; heavy shoes; large nails; and nails set too far back. Cracks which start at the bottom are usually due to shoeing and are of little importance, while those that start at the coronet are usually troublesome.

Symptoms —A crack in the wall at the toe or the quarter. The crack may be shallow and cause no lameness, or it may extend entirely through the wall, injuring the sensitive structures within.

Treatment.—Remove the shoe and soften the horn by foot baths or poultices. This being accomplished, cut away the overlapping edges of the crack and thin the horn on each side. A bar shoe is then applied, the wall beneath the crack being cut away so that it will not come in contact with the shoe. A cantharides blister should then be applied to the coronet above the crack to stimulate a new growth of horn. Toe cracks are treated in the same way.

456. Contracted feet.—An unnatural narrowing of the feet at the quarters and heels. Most frequently seen in the front feet.

Causes.—Lack of frog pressure; lack of exercise; excessive dryness of the feet; concaving of the bearing surface of the shoe back to the heels; cutting away the bars, and opening the heels with the knife.

Symptoms.—The foot, instead of being wide at the quarters and circular in shape, becomes narrow at the heels, which in very severe cases may overlap. The frog atrophies and is often affected with thrush. Lameness may be present as a result of the pinching of the sensitive structures by the walls of the hoof.

Treatment—Frog pressure is essential. This may be obtained by the use of a bar shoe, with leather pad, tar, and oakum, or by letting the animal run barefoot for several months on soft ground. Faults in shoeing must be corrected. If the foot is hard and dry it must be softened by soaking or poulticing.

457. Dry feet.—A troublesome condition occurring most frequently in dry weather.

Causes.—Lack of exercise; lack of frog pressure; dry weather; and rasping away the periople.

Symptoms.—A hard, dry, and inelastic condition of the horn. This increases concussion and frequently causes inflammation of the foot corium and produces lameness.

Treatment—Soften the feet by poultices or by foot baths and then apply an oily covering to the wall surface; or, pack the cavity between the branches of the shoe with wet clay two or three times a week. This is preferable to soaking in water as it supplies moisture to the foot and does not macerate the periople. Work the animal on soft ground whenever possible. Oils and ointments do not soften the hoof. They are only useful to prevent drying out after the foot has been moistened.

458. Navicular disease.—A chronic inflammation at the point where the tendon of the deep digital flexor passes over the navicular bone. The disease is confined almost exclusively to the front feet and to light horses and mules used for fast work.

Causes.—Concussion; violent strains thrown upon the deep flexor tendon; improper preparation of the foot in shoeing—i. e., leaving the toe too long or excessive lowering of the heels.

Symptoms.—In the early stages there is little to indicate the nature of the disease. There is lameness which may be slight at first, but which gradually increases in severity. When resting the animal points the toe, and if lame in both feet the limbs are advanced and the feet rested alternately. In traveling the affected leg takes a short step and the toe strikes the ground before the heel comes down. In some cases the lameness may disappear for a day or two, but only to return with greater severity than ever. At times there is increased sensitiveness of the foot, and pressure over the navicular area with the tester causes great pain. Bar shoes greatly increase the lameness. As time goes on the frog atrophies, the heels contract, and the wall at the heel becomes higher than normal.

Treatment.—The disease is incurable and only relief can be given. In the early stages reduce the inflammation with cold baths or cold packs. The toe is then carefully shortened and a shoe with a rolled toe and thickened heels applied. The foot should be softened two or three times a week by means of foot baths or poultices and a light coating of *linseed oil* or *cosmoline* applied.

When possible the animal should be allowed to run barefoot on soft ground for several months.

459. Punctured wounds of the frog and sole—Pricks in shoeing.

Causes.—Punctures of the frog and sole are caused by the animal stepping on nails, pieces of glass, sharp sticks, and other pointed objects.

Pricks in shoeing may be *direct* or *indirect*.

In *direct* pricking the nail is driven directly into the sensitive structures, causing immediate lameness.

In *indirect* pricking the nail is not driven into the sensitive tissues, but so close that it crowds the inner layer of the horn in against them. In such cases lameness may not appear for several days.

Symptoms.—Lameness more or less severe. The foot is hot; there is more or less throbbing in the digital arteries, and pressure with the tester over the injured spot causes pain. If the animal goes lame immediately after having been shod, pricking is to be suspected. Clean the foot thoroughly, remove the nails one at a time and examine each nail carefully for moisture, blood, or pus. Test each nail hole with the tester or pincers; when the injured spot is pressed, the horse will flinch. If the nails are found to have produced no injury examine the frog and the rest of the sole in the same manner for nails or other sharp objects that may have been picked up in the road or elsewhere.

Treatment.—Whether old or recent, whether caused by pricking or by a nail or other sharp object, the treatment is the same   Trim the horn carefully from about the wound, remove the offending object if present, and establish drainage. Clean the wound thoroughly with a strong antiseptic solution; dry it well with clean cotton and apply *tincture of iodine*. The foot is then well bandaged and the animal placed in a clean, dry stall. Repeat the dressings twice daily until pus formation and lameness cease. The wound is then packed with tar and oakum and the horse shod as directed in paragraph 453.

460. Quittor.—A chronic inflammation of the cartilages of the foot and their surrounding structures, characterized by the presence of one or more small openings (fistulas) from which there is a continuous discharge of pus.

Causes—Treads on the coronet, suppurating corns, and bruised and punctured wounds of the sole.

Symptoms.—Heat, swelling, and tenderness in the region of the coronet and heel, usually the inner one. The inflammation may subside, but usually an abscess forms and discharges a bloody pus, after which the swelling may disappear, leaving one or more small canals (fistulas, sinuses) 1 or 2 inches in depth. There is usually lameness.

Treatment.—Rest. If due to a nail wound, a tread or a suppurating corn, treat accordingly. The canals may be injected twice daily with *tincture of iodine* and a pack of a 1 to 1,000 solution of *bichloride of mercury applied*. If this does not affect a cure, an operation will be necessary.

461. Seedy toe.—A mealy condition of the horn of the wall, usually in the region of the toe.

Causes—Usually results from an attack of laminitis. Excessive moisture is also said to be a cause

Symptoms—A crumbling and breaking away of the white line between the wall and the sole, leading to the formation of a hollow wall. By tapping on the wall of the diseased part a hollow sound may be heard.

Treatment.—Scrape out the soft, crumbly horn and clean the cavity well; apply *tincture of iodine* or *pure creolin* and pack with *tar* and *oakum*. The foot is then shod with a leather pad and a bar shoe. A cantharides blister should be applied to the coronet to stimulate the growth of the horn.

462. Thrush.—A disease of the frog characterized by an offensive odor and a softening of the horn.

Causes.—Muddy roads, picket lines and corrals, and a filthy condition of the floor of the stables in which the animal is kept.

Symptoms.—A stinking discharge from the cleft of the frog. As the disease advances the discharge and odor become more marked, the cleft deepens, the horn becomes underrun and loosened, and the sensitive structures are exposed. Lameness is uaually absent, it occurring only in severe cases, where the whole or a large portion of the frog is diseased.

Treatment.—Clean, dry stalls are essential. Pare away all loose underrun portions of horn, dry-clean the frog thoroughly with oakum and apply *tincture of iodine*. When the iodine dries, cover the parts with *pine tar*. Or, after the frog has been thoroughly cleaned, pack with the *three sulphates*, or a few drops of *pure creolin*. If not lame, keep the animal at work.

463. Treads.—Injuries of the coronet and heels.

Causes.—Stepping with the shoe of one foot upon the coronet or heel of another in turning, backing, or going to one side, and sometimes by a tread from another horse. Cavalry horses and lead and swing horses of artillery are often injured by the horses in rear when column is brought suddenly to a halt.

Symptoms.—Laceration or bruising, with heat, pain, and swelling in the region of the heels or coronet.

Treatment.—Remove all portions of loosened horn and treat as directed in paragraphs 353 and 357.

CHAPTER XVII.

ISOLATION, QUARANTINE, AND DISINFECTION.

ISOLATION.

464. Isolation is a preventative measure wherein an animal affected with a contagious disease, or one suspected of such a disease, is separated from the healthy animals and placed by itself. To be effective, isolation must be complete, otherwise it is useless. In summer or in the Tropics, in order to prevent the spreading of disease by flies, diseased animals should be removed to a place at least 200 or 300 yards from the healthy ones and kept within an inclosure having preferably a double fence, the fences to be separated by a space of 10 or 12 feet to avoid all possibility of contact with animals which may be on the outside. In winter, the distance between the sick and healthy need not be so great.

Each isolated animal must be provided with a separate feed box, water bucket, blanket, and grooming outfit, none of which should be removed from the place of isolation until properly disinfected. Only authorized persons should be permitted to enter the place of isolation. Attendants should have no duties which bring them in contact with other animals. They should wear fatigue clothing, and on leaving the place of isolation this clothing should be removed, the hands and face washed with soap and water, and the hands and shoes disinfected. The fatigue clothing should not be removed from the place of isolation until thoroughly disinfected.

No animal, carcass, forage, bedding, or manure should be removed from the place of isolation without proper authority. As the dung, nasal discharges, etc., of an infected animal often contain the germs of disease, they, together with all soiled bedding, hay, grain, etc., should be piled up within the corral, saturated with crude oil, and burned, and disinfectants used freely about the stall. This procedure is not only of value in the destruction of infectious material, but also in destroying the breeding places of flies.

Immediately after an animal has been removed from the stable and placed in isolation, his entire equipment, his stall, the watering trough, the salt boxes, and everything used upon him, and everything with which he has been in contact, should be thoroughly disinfected.

157

465. Diseases for which animals should be isolated:
Eczema (Dhobie itch).
Epizootic lymphangitis.
Glanders.
Influenza.
Lice.
Mange.
Nasal catarrh of whatever nature.
Pneumonia.
Ringworm.
Strangles.
Surra.

QUARANTINE.

466. By quarantine is meant the period during which animals suffering from contagious disease are kept away from those known to be healthy. It also means the detention and isolation of animals coming from places infected, or suspected of being infected, with contagious disease. There is no fixed period of quarantine for all cases, but the length of this period varies according to the nature of the disease against which the quarantine is established. As a general rule it should be at least ten days or two weeks in length. Animals, particularly remounts, should be quarantined upon their arrival at camp or garrison to determine whether or not they have been exposed to diseases of contagious or infectious nature.

To be of value quarantine must be perfect, otherwise it is as useless as none at all. Not only should the diseased animals themselves be quarantined against, but also all animals, stables, equipment, etc., which may have been exposed to the infection.

During the period of quarantine all animals showing symptoms of contagious disease should be segregated immediately in different isolated places, and their stalls, together with their feeding, watering, and grooming utensils, thoroughly disinfected. The remaining animals must then be held for another period of 10 days or 2 weeks.

Quarantine pens or corrals should be at least 200 or 300 yards from all susceptible animals.

For quarantinable diseases see paragraph 465.

DISINFECTION.

467. By this term is meant the destruction of organisms causing contagious and infectious diseases. This may be accomplished by means of *sunlight* and *heat* or by the use of *chemical agents*

468. Sunlight.—Germs of many diseases will live almost indefinitely in dark, damp places, while in the sunlight they exist only for a short time.

469. Heat.—(a) For the destruction of material contaminated with germs of disease, such as manure, nasal discharges, soiled forage and bedding, and worthless articles of equipment, there is nothing more convenient and more certain than the application of fire. When burning of such material is conducted in the open air, great care must be taken that the burning is complete and that no small unburned particles remain to be scattered about by the action of the wind. To insure thoroughness in burning, saturate the material to be burned with crude oil or kerosene.

(b) Boiling for 20 minutes is an effective method for the destruction of disease-producing germs. Its use, however, is limited to articles of a metallic or earthen nature and to clothing, etc., of linen or cotton. Articles of wool (blankets) or leather must not be boiled.

470. Chemical agents.—The chemical agents most frequently used in disinfection are:

To 1 gallon of water—

Bichloride of mercury	drams..	2
Carbolic acid	ounces..	6½
Chloride of lime (fresh)	do....	6
Chloro naptholeum	do....	4
Creolin	do....	4
Formalin	do....	6
Kreso	do....	4
Liquor cresolis	do....	5

471. Disinfection of stables.—Entire stables or individual stalls are disinfected after the removal of the occupants and the isolation of the sick. The method of procedure is as follows:

Feed boxes and mangers should be thoroughly cleaned and the bedding and manure removed from the stalls and piled up outside. The walls, floors, and partitions should then be scraped and swept clean and the sweepings placed on the pile with the bedding and burned. If the floor be of earth, three or four inches of the surface should be dug up and removed to some place inaccessible to live stock and saturated with a good disinfectant. The removed earth should be replaced with clean, fresh, uncontaminated clay. Should any of the woodwork about the stable have become softened or decayed it should be removed, burned, and replaced with new material.

The stable having been carefully cleaned, the disinfectant, preferably creolin, kreso, or bichloride of mercury, is then applied thoroughly to all surfaces, such as walls, partitions, mangers, and floors (if of concrete or brick). This may be accomplished by the use of brooms or brushes, but the best and most efficient method is by means of a strong spray pump with which the disinfecting solution can be forced into all cracks and crevices. The walls and posts should be disinfected to a height of at least 12 feet from the floor. Feed boxes, and mangers should receive particular attention. The corral should be cleaned thoroughly, and the watering trough, fences, picket lines, and salt boxes thoroughly disinfected. The process of disinfection having been completed, the stable or stall is allowed to dry for three or four days before again being used. When the entire stable has been disinfected, it is well to open all doors and windows for the admission of air and light.

When disinfection follows an outbreak of mange the stable should not be reoccupied within 8 or 10 days. A second disinfection 6 or 8 days after the first is also advisable. In this case unslacked lime may be added to the disinfecting solution. In the Tropics, infected stables constructed of bamboo and other cheap material should be burned.

472. Disinfection of leather.—Bridles, halters, and harnesses should be taken apart, and the stirrups, coat straps, etc , removed from the saddle. All parts are then given a thorough scrubbing with warm water, soap, and a stiff brush, after which they are allowed to dry. They should then be scrubbed with a solution of creolin, kreso, liquor cresolis, or carbolic acid, and dried. The drying in both cases should take place in the shade.

473. Disinfection of blankets and grooming utensils.—Such articles are best disinfected by placing them for 12 hours in a bath of creolin, kreso, bichloride of mercury, liquor cresolis, or carbolic acid.

474. Disinfection of men's clothing.—Articles of wool should be soaked for 12 hours as directed in paragraph 473. Articles of linen or cotton should be boiled or soaked in a disinfectant.

475. Disinfection of bits, curbchains, and other like articles of metal.—Boil or scrub well with any of the disinfectants except bichloride of mercury, which will corrode them.

476. Disinfection of stable implements.—Forks, brooms, buckets, etc., should be freed from dirt, scrubbed with soap and water, and washed with a disinfectant.

477. Disinfection of watering troughs, feed boxes, etc.— Scrub with boiling water and soap, then wash thoroughly with a disinfectant

478. Disinfection of railroad cars.—Cars are disinfected in the same manner as stables.

DESTRUCTION OF ANIMALS.

479. Destruction of animals is best accomplished by shooting with a pistol. An imaginary line is drawn from the base of the right ear to the left eye and vice versa. The bullet should enter at the point where these two lines cross, the pistol being held close to the head.

DISPOSAL OF CARCASSES

480. By burning.—Dig a trench in the ground in the shape of a cross (+), each trench being 7 feet long, 15 inches wide, and 18 inches deep at the point where the two meet, becoming shallower at each end. The earth is thrown up in the angles formed by the trench, and on this are placed two stout pieces of iron (a piece of railroad rail if obtainable) or wooden rails. A layer of stout wood is placed on the rails, and on this the carcass is placed. Wood is then piled over the carcass and the pile lighted with paper, straw, shavings, etc. Five gallons of crude oil or kerosene poured over the carcass will hasten the burning. The carcass is usually consumed in five or six hours. Blood, manure, nasal discharges, etc., which may be scattered about on the ground, should be scraped up with the earth and thrown into the fire.

481. By burying.—When burning is impracticable, carcasses should be buried. The grave should be at least 8 feet deep and the carcass should be well covered with unslacked lime, after which the grave is filled in and the earth well packed. Earth which has been soiled by blood, manure, nasal discharges, etc , should be scraped up and thrown into the bottom of the grave.

Wagons, etc , in which animals dead of contagious disease are hauled should be cleaned and disinfected.

Flies.

482. Flies.—In addition to their importance on account of the worry produced by their bites and the loss of blood suffered by their victims, flies are of great importance as carriers of disease. For these reasons their destruction as well as the destruction of the material in which they breed must receive constant and vigilant attention.

483. Breeding places of flies.—Flies breed principally in horse manure, damp straw or hay, fallen leaves, dead grass, underbrush, decaying animal and vegetable matter, refuse and filth of every kind, and in earth soaked with horse urine.

484. Control of flies in garrison.—During fly season, or in the Tropics, the stables must be kept absolutely clean and dry. Manure, soiled bedding, and refuse about the feed boxes and mangers should be removed daily and hauled to the dump. Food boxes and mangers should be swept or brushed out daily, and once a week the feed boxes and a portion of the woodwork immediately surrounding them should be well scraped and washed clean with boiling water. The doors and windows should be kept open at all times, except during storms, and bales of hay or straw, and empty sacks or sacks filled with grain that may have become wet by rain blowing through open windows or doors should be scattered about and allowed to dry.

The corrals and picket lines should be swept daily, and special attention must be paid to the ground beneath the watering trough to see that it is kept clean and dry. If the floor of the picket line should be of soft earth, it should be sprinkled once a week with crude oil.

Horse covers and saddle blankets that have been used and which for any reason are to be stored away in the stable should be thoroughly dried before storing.

485. Fly traps and fly poison.—These are often useful in the destruction of flies, particularly in and about stables. An excellent fly poison is made as follows:

Formalin................................ounce..	1
Sugar or sirup.............................do....	1
Water.......................................pint..	1

Mix. Put in shallow vessels and place where the flies are the thickest.

486. Control of flies in camp.—When animals are to remain in camp for more than a few days, the picket lines and the ground for 50 yards or more on the sides and ends should be thoroughly

policed. Underbrush, tall grass, etc., should be cut and burned
or removed to an out-of-the-way place several hundred yards from
the camp. The floor of the picket line and the ground for several
feet on either side should be raked and swept daily, and the manure,
straw, and other sweepings burned or hauled away to the camp
dump. Once a week the floor of the picket line should be burned
with crude oil and straw at the rate of 10 gallons of crude oil and 75
pounds of straw to each line.

The accumulation of waste and filth from any source must not be
permitted, and bales of hay or straw and empty sacks and sacks of
grain that may have become wet should be scattered about in the
sun to dry. Loose straw or hay should be treated in the same way.

487. Protection of animals against bites of flies.—External
applications for this purpose are not satisfactory, although many
have been tried. Sick horses and horses in isolation may be kept
in screened stalls or covered with gunny sacking or other light
material.

CHAPTER XVIII.

CONTAGIOUS AND INFECTIOUS DISEASES.

488. Contagious and infectious diseases are diseases capable of being transmitted from one animal to another. They are caused by germs, fungi, and low forms of animal life.

Animals affected, or suspected of being affected, with a contagious disease should be isolated at once in a well-ventilated place and all places to which they have had access thoroughly disinfected. Particular attention should be given to all drinking and feeding utensils, especially those which are to be used by other animals. A veterinarian should be notified at once in all cases where such a disease is suspected.

489. Contagious stomatitis (figs. 50, 51).—A mild contagious inflammation of the mucous membrane of the mouth, involving sometimes the mucous membrane of the nose and the skin of the lips

Cause.—The cause is unknown. The disease is spread by the saliva of the sick which contaminates the food and water of other animals. It is also spread by the hands of attendants, grooming utensils, etc.

Symptoms.—The animal takes its food slowly and chews with great care, and there is always more or less slobbering, the saliva hanging from the mouth in long threads. The animal holds the mouth shut. If opened, a quantity of saliva spills out. The mucous membrane of the mouth is reddened, and the lips and cheeks are often swollen and tender. On the mucous membrane of the lips, gums, tongue, roof of the mouth, and beneath the tongue appear hard, red elevations about the size of a pea, from which, in a few days, little blisters are formed. Sometimes small abscesses are formed, which break and leave behind small round ulcers. These ulcers and blisters usually heal in five or six days, leaving behind a white scar. The lump is usually slightly elevated.

The disease usually ends in recovery in about two weeks.

Treatment.—Feed soft food and allow plenty of fresh drinking water. Wash out the mouth three times a day with *creolin* 4 drams, water 1 pint; or, *potassium permanganate* 30 grains to 1 quart of water.

490. Strangles (distemper).—An acute contagious and infectious disease of horses and mules, occurring most commonly in animals from 6 months to 5 years of age.

Cause. —A germ, the streptococcus equi.

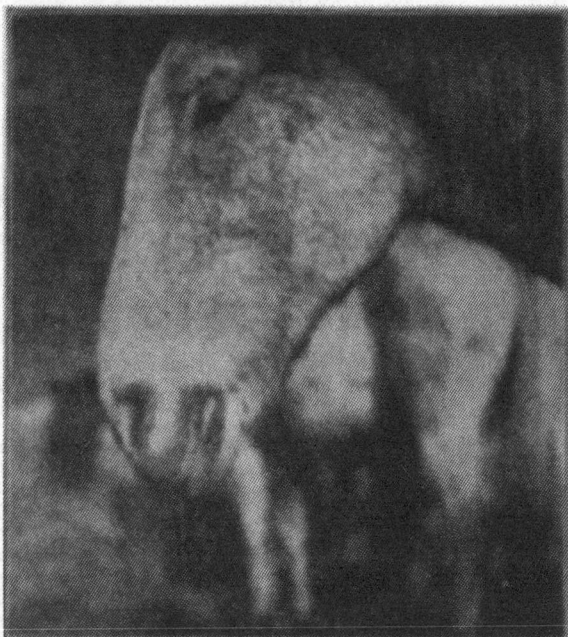

FIG. 50.—Contagious stomatitis. (By courtesy of Dr. S. Stewart.)

Symptoms.—The disease begins with a high fever, ranging from 104° to 106°; and an abundant discharge from the nose which is at first watery, but later becomes much thicker. The submaxillary glands (the glands below the lower jaw) swell, become hot and painful, and in them abscesses may form. There is soreness of the throat, cough, loss of appetite, depression, and occasionally great muscular weakness. There may be some swelling of the limbs and occasionally swellings are found elsewhere on the body. The infection may spread along the lymph channels and cause blood poisoning and death.

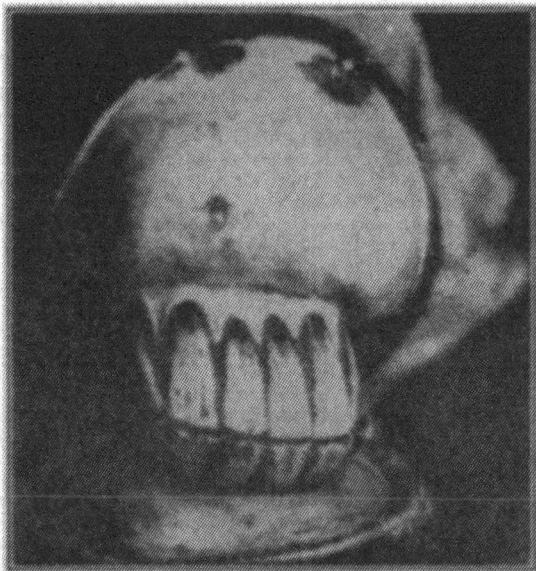

Fig. 51.—Contagious stomatitis. (By courtesy of Dr. S. Stewart.)

Treatment.—Clothe the body according to the season; avoid drafts; apply stimulating liniments, hot baths, or poultices to the enlarged glands three times a day, and, as soon as a soft area is noticed, open and flush twice daily with an antiseptic solution. (See Abscess, par. 372.)

Feed soft foods, such as grass, bran mashes, steamed oats. Supply an abundance of fresh drinking water to which has been added one-half ounce of *potassium nitrate* two or three times a day. During convalescence give moderate exercise, tonics, and plenty of grain.

491. Influenza (pinkeye, catarrhal fever).—An acute contagious and infectious disease affecting the respiratory and digestive mucous membranes, the eyes, and the nervous and circulatory systems.

Cause.—An organism the nature of which little is known.

Symptoms.—The first symptoms noticed are loss of appetite, depression, and great weakness. The animal staggers when walking, the head is held low, and the temperature rises to 105° or 107°. The eyes are often intensely inflamed and the visible mucous membranes become yellowish in color. There is often a discharge from the nostrils, which may be watery at first, but later becomes thicker and often tinged with yellow. Respiration is quickened, and when the digestive organs are affected colic may occur. At first there is constipation and the dung is coated with a thin layer of mucus. Later, diarrhea may set in and the legs may become swollen, hot, and sensitive to the touch. During the course of the disease pneumonia sometimes develops.

Treatment.—Absolute rest. Clothe the body according to the season; provide plenty of fresh drinking water and give soft food, except when diarrhea exists, in which case give hay, dry bran, oatmeal, or crushed oats. Colic may be relieved by giving *cannabis indica, fluid extract of belladonna*, or the *camphor* and *carbolic acid* preparation as prescribed in paragraph 414. Give one-half ounce doses of *potassium nitrate* in drinking water two or three times daily. *Quinine sulphate* may be given twice a day in 1-dram doses. If great weakness is in evidence, combine the *quinine* with 1 dram *fluid extract of nux vomica* and give twice daily. Or, give *alcohol* or *spirits of nitrous ether* in 2 to 4 ounce doses three times daily in the drinking water.

The eyes, if involved, should be treated as directed in paragraph 435. Should pneumonia develop, treat as directed in paragraph 422. Animals should not be worked for at least two weeks after the temperature has become normal.

During an outbreak of influenza in a stable early morning temperatures should be taken daily. Any animal showing increase of temperature should be isolated.

492. Contagious pneumonia (pleuropneumonia, infectious pneumonia).—An acute contagious and infectious disease affecting the lungs and pleuræ. Although rather slow in spreading from animal to animal, it often causes great losses when once introduced into a stable.

Cause.—Not yet identified.

Symptoms and treatment.—The same as for pneumonia. (See par. 422.)

During an outbreak of contagious pneumonia in a stable early morning temperatures should be taken daily. Any animal showing increase of temperature should be isolated.

493. Glanders.—A contagious and infectious disease, which may be transmitted to man. It may be *acute* or *chronic*. The external form of the disease is called *farcy*.

Cause.—The bacillus of glanders.

494. Acute glanders (fig. 52) —This form is most common in the mule, though it may occur in horses while in transit and in tropical climates.

Symptoms.—Chill; temperature, 105° to 107°; discharge from the nose, which may be bloody; pimples and ulcers on the mucous membrane of the nostrils, which sometimes perforate the nasal septum; respirations quickened and often difficult; rapid emaciation; and great weakness. Later, diarrhea may occur. The lymph glands of the lower jaw become enlarged and nodules and ulcers may form in the skin. The course of this form is rapid and death takes place in from 3 to 14 days.

Treatment.—None. (See par. 496.)

495. Chronic glanders.—This is the form most frequently seen in the horse in temperate climates.

Symptoms.—The first symptom noticed is usually a discharge from one or both nostrils, which is whitish in color and which may later become tinged with blood. Pimples form on the mucous membrane of the nostrils and soon change to ulcers, which are more or less deep and have thickened and ragged edges. These ulcers frequently cause small hemorrhages and the nasal discharge then becomes mixed with blood. The submaxillary lymph glands become slightly thickened and sensitive, but later they become knotlike and pain-less. The animal becomes weak, emaciated, and easily fatigued. Cough and more or less interference with breathing may be noticed. The temperature may be slightly elevated and irregular. The progress of the disease is slow and the animal may live for years. In some cases prominent symptoms never develop during the life of the animal

Treatment.—None. (See par. 496)

496. Farcy (skin glanders).—This is most commonly seen as a symptom of acute glanders.

Symptoms.—Nodules, the size of a pea to that of a walnut, appear, as a rule, on the shoulders, neck, chest, and limbs. The superficial

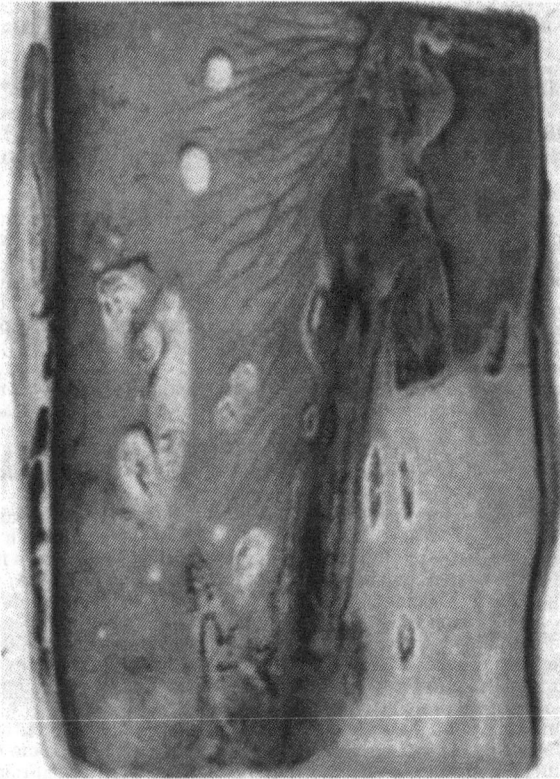

FIG. 52.—GLANDERS.

Middle region of nasal septum, left side, showing ulcers. (From "Diseases of the Horse," Department of Agriculture.)

lymphatics become enlarged and appear as knotted cords, and in them ulcers discharging a sticky, bloody fluid are formed. The ulcers heal but slowly, if at all, leaving behind small jagged scars.

Treatment.—None. The disease is incurable. The affected animal should be destroyed at once and burned and the stables and all equipment thoroughly disinfected. All exposed animals in the organization and post should be quarantined and repeatedly

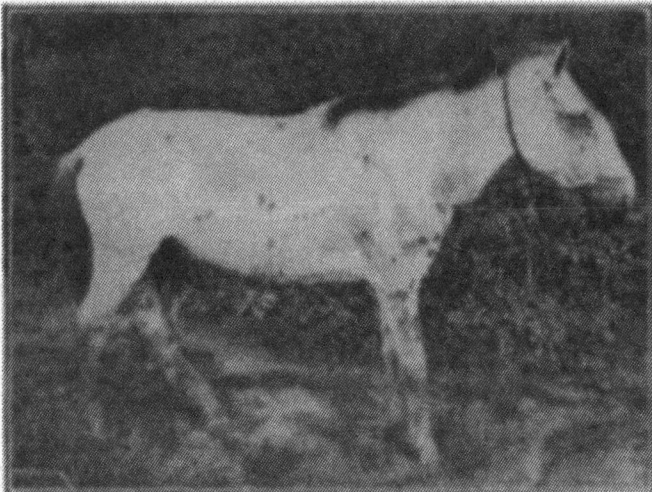

Fig. 53.—Chronic epizootic lymphangitis (tropical).

tested with one or more of the various tests until all are proven to be free from the disease. All animals which react to the test should be destroyed. These tests can be carried out only by a veterinarian.

497. Epizootic lymphangitis (figs. 53, 54).—A chronic, contagious disease which spreads slowly through the lymphatic vessels and lymphatic glands. It is somewhat similar to *farcy* (skin glanders), except that in the latter there may be rise of temperature and sudden loss of flesh and vigor which are not seen in *epizootic lymphangitis.*

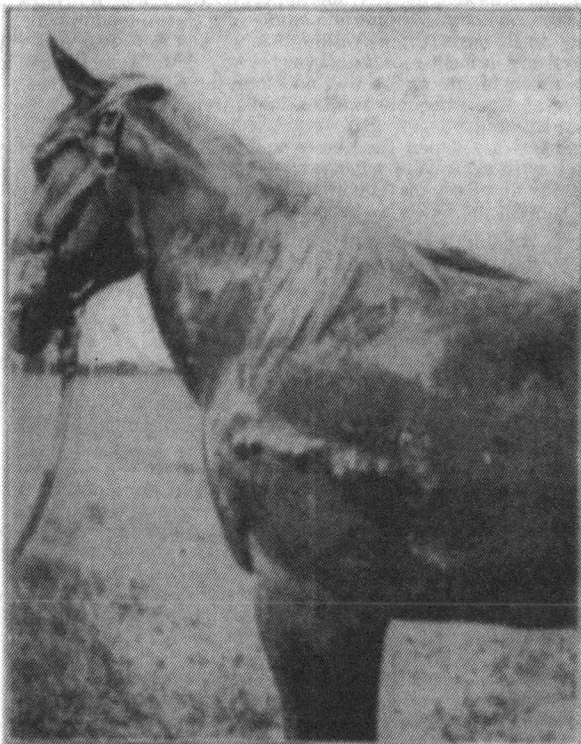

Fig. 54.—Chronic epizootic lymphangitis (tropical)

Cause.—A fungus.

Symptoms.—Nodules, either singly or in clusters, or in the form of a string of beads, usually first appear on the limbs, but later on any part of the body. From the nodules abscesses develop, which break and discharge a thick, yellow pus. When the abscesses rupture, ulcers are formed, which heal very slowly. In cases of long standing the ulcers often run together and form large ulcerous surfaces. The infected limbs become swollen, and the patient becomes weak and poor in flesh.

Treatment.—Open the abscesses, clean them out thoroughly, and pack with crystals of *potassium permanganate* or *sulphate of copper*. Or, the abscesses may be swabbed out and the ulcers painted once daily with the following caustic solution:

Bichloride of mercury	drams..	2
Salicylic acid	ounces..	1
Alcohol	do....	4

Mix. Apply with a small cotton swab. When pus ceases, apply ordinary antiseptics.

As the disease is frequently spread by flies, the ulcers should be covered or treated as directed in paragraph 360. The manure, soiled bedding, and all cast-off dressings and bandages should be burned. All instruments, etc., used about the patient must be thoroughly disinfected.

498. Tetanus (lockjaw) (fig. 55)—An infectious disease caused by a germ which is found in the soil, in manure, and in manured ground (gardens, around stables). The germ enters the body through wounds, and animals sustaining deep punctured wounds which become soiled with earth or manure are likely to develop the disease. Punctured wounds of the feet are especially dangerous. The germ does not readily grow in large open wounds, because in such wounds oxygen (air) is freely admitted. It is more prevalent in hot than in cold climates.

Cause.—The bacillus of tetanus.

Symptoms.—Usually develop in one or two days. The first symptom noticed is a slight general muscular stiffness interfering with movement, mastication, swallowing, and drinking. Slight muscular spasms may also be noticed. In a short time the stiffness increases; the head is held extended; the tail is elevated, and the ears are held erect. Prehension and mastication become more and more difficult or impossible, and food and saliva collect in the mouth and decompose. The muscles become firmly contracted and hard; the jaws are set; the nostrils are dilated, and the limbs are greatly

stiffened and stand well apart. If forced to move, the legs are carried like stilts with little or no bending of the joints. There is
muscular twitching and excitement, both of which are increased
by any sudden noise, a flash of light, or a slap of the hand.

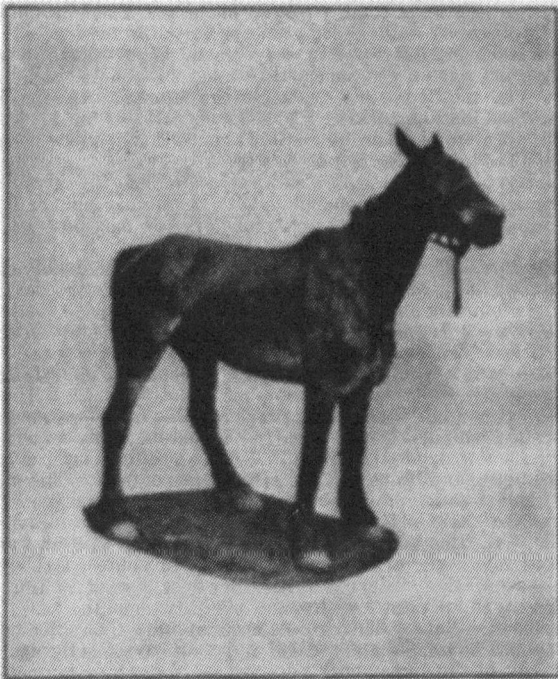

FIG. 55.—Tetanus.

The eye is drawn well into its socket and the haw (membrana
nictitans) partially covers the eyeball. There may be profuse
sweating. The temperature is at first normal or slightly elevated.
Later it may rise to 105° or over.

In cases which develop quickly death may occur in from one to three days, the average duration of fatal cases being about one week. Recovery is seldom complete in less than four or five weeks. The mortality is from 80 to 85 per cent.

Treatment.—If the wound can be found, open it well and treat with an antiseptic, preferably *tincture* of *iodine*. Place the animal in a quiet, darkened stall. Feed gruels or very thin mashes, and keep fresh water constantly within easy reach. The vessels in which the food and water are given should be supported at a height of 3 or 4 feet from the floor—this to enable the animal to eat and drink without bending the neck.

Medicines are of little use. Give from 2 to 4 ounces *potassium bromide* in the drinking water twice a day; or ½-ounce doses of *cannabis indica* in one pint of warm water may be given as an enema and repeated often enough to keep the animal quiet or drowsy. Do not attempt to drench or give balls. Slings *may* be used when necessary to keep the animal on its feet.

Prevention.—The disease may be prevented by thoroughly cleansing all wounds, expecially punctured wounds of the feet, and treating them with antiseptics.

499. Surra (fig. 56).—A tropical contagious and infectious blood disease, transmitted by biting insects, especially flies.

Cause.—A low form of animal life, the trypanosoma evansi (fig. 57).

Symptoms —Dullness, depression, and great weakness. The temperature rises from 104° to 106°, and remains high for four or five days, after which it may return to the normal, only to shoot up again in a few days. Later, soft, doughy swellings appear on the sheath, belly, and limbs. There is rapid loss of flesh. The mucous membranes become pale and frequently show dark red spots (petechiae), and there may be a watery discharge from the eyes and nostrils. The temperature continues to rise and fall, the animal becomes more and more emaciated, and, in acute cases, dies in about two weeks. The disease is, however, usually chronic, in which case the patient may live for one or two months.

Treatment.—None. The disease is incurable. The affected animals should be immediately killed and their carcasses burned.

To prevent the spread of the disease, early morning temperatures of all the animals in the post or camp should be taken daily. Any animal showing a rise of temperature should be isolated. His temperature should be taken daily and a veterinarian should examine his blood. The suspected animal should be protected from flies either by being placed in a screened building or by being covered with sacking or a net. Every effort should be made to destroy flies

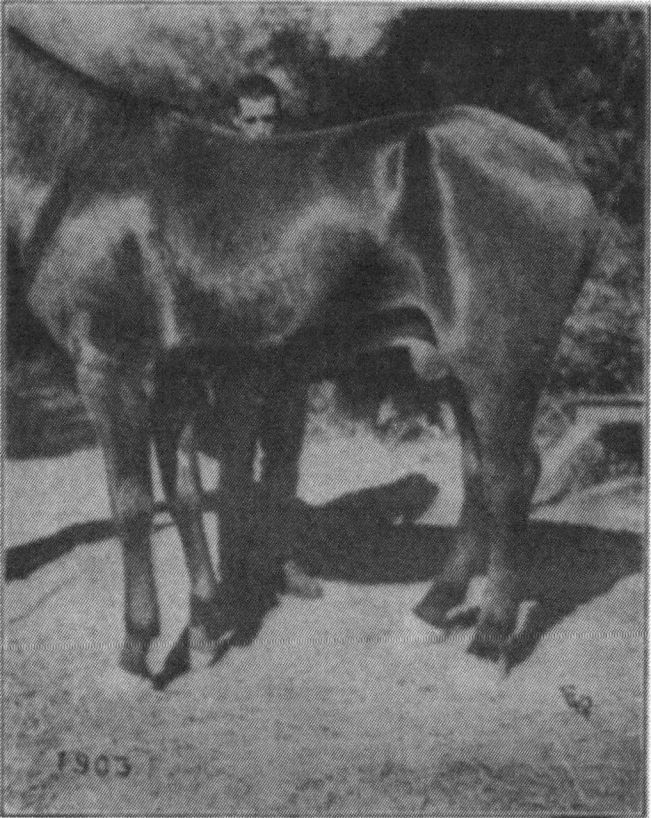

FIG. 56.—Surra; characteristic swellings.

and prevent their breeding. Cattle and carabao may carry the infection. They should therefore be excluded from the post or camp.

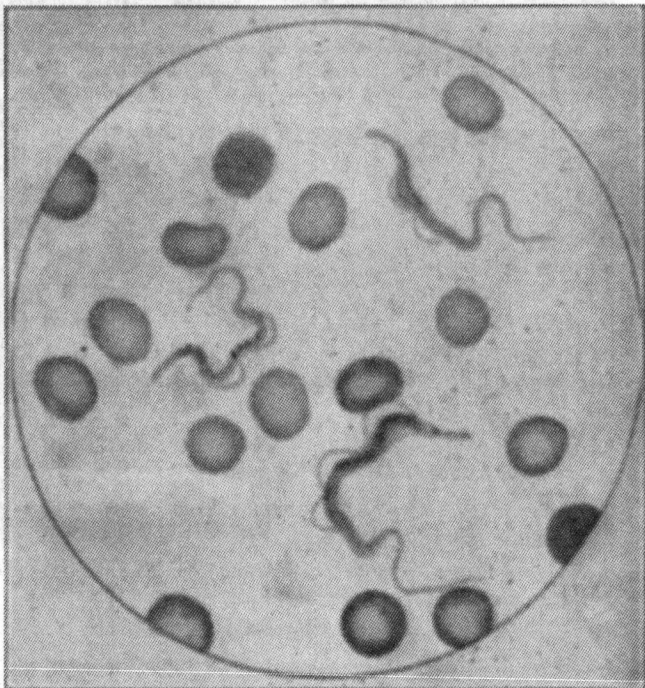

Fig. 57 —Trypanosoma evansi (the worm-like figures).

500. Purpura hemorrhagica (purpura, petechial fever) (fig. 58).—An acute noncontagious disease of horses and mules. It may

106233°—17——12

occur independently, but usually follows such diseases as strangles, pneumonia, and influenza.

Cause.—Unknown

Symptoms.—On the mucous membranes of the nostrils and eyes there appear small, dark red spots, varying in size from that of a pin's head to a pea. At about the same time swellings appear on the head, belly, and legs, which become enormous in size. These swellings have a characteristic abruptly terminating border, giving

FIG. 58.—Purpura hemorrhagica.

the appearance of having been tied with a string. The swellings of the legs cause stiffness, and the swellings of the head and nostrils may become so great as to interfere with breathing. The temperature is at first normal, but may become elevated in a few days.

Treatment.—There is no specific. Tie the head up high. Give easily digested food and tonics. If the swellings break open or crack, apply antiseptics. If suffocation threatens, bathe nostrils with cold water. *Tincture* of *chloride* of *iron* is probably the best tonic. It should be given twice a day.

GLOSSARY.

Abdomen: The cavity between the thorax and the pelvis.

Abscess: A collection of pus.

Absorb: Take in, suck up, take up.

Absorption: The taking in of fluids or other substances by the skin, mucous surfaces, or absorbent vessels.

Acute: Having a short, severe course; not chronic.

Adjust: Put in order, arrange, set to rights.

Anterior: Situated in front of or in the forward part of.

Aqueous: Watery; prepared with water.

Arm: The region between the shoulder and forearm.

Articular: Pertaining to a joint.

Ascend: Rise, climb, go up.

Atrophy: A wasting or diminution in the size of a part.

Auxiliary: That which affords aid.

Bacillus: Rod-shaped germ.

Bacterium (bacteria, plural): A germ.

Barrel: The body or trunk.

Base: The lowest part or foundation of anything.

Basis: The base or lower part.

Bog: Soft and spongy.

Bowel· The intestine.

Brain: The mass of nervous material within the cranium.

Buttocks: The protuberances of the rump on either side of the tail.

Canal: Any tube, narrow passage, or channel.

Canine: Of or pertaining to, or like that which belongs to a dog.

Cannon: The structures between the knee (hock in hind leg) and the fetlock.

Capricious: Odd, queer, freakish, uncertain, changeable.

Cartilage: Gristle.

Catarrh: Inflammation of a mucous membrane, with a free discharge.

Caudal: Pertaining to the tail.

Cecum (cæcum): Blind; blind gut.

Chestnuts: The horny plates found on the inside of the legs near the knee and hock; so called on account of their fanciful resemblance to a chestnut.

Chronic: Long continued; not acute.

Clot: A soft mass of coagulated blood or lymph.

177

Coagulate: To curdle; thicken; clot.

Coma: Profound stupor.

Compress: A pad of any kind, applied so as to make pressure on any particular part.

Concave: Hollow, depressed, hollowed out.

Concussion: A violent jar or shock.

Conformation: Structure, form, shape.

Congestion: An excess of blood in a part.

Constipation: Infrequent evacuation of the bowel.

Contagion: The communication of disease by contact, either direct or indirect; a contagious disease.

Contagious: Carried from one person or animal to another; catching.

Contraction: A shortening.

Convalescence: The stage of recovery following an attack of disease.

Convalescent: A patient in the stage of recovery following an attack of disease.

Convex: Bulging, rounding outwardly.

Coronet: A crown; the crown of the hoof.

Corpuscles: Small cells which form part of the blood.

Corrode: Eat away, consume, impair, destroy

Corrosive: Destructive to tissue, caustic, eating away.

Coxa: The hip or hip bone.

Cranium: The skull or brain pan.

Croup: That portion of the upper part of the body situated between the loins in front and the tail behind.

Crystalline: Resembling a crystal.

Dandruff: Scales found upon the skin.

Debilitating: Weakening.

Descend: To go down.

Decomposition: Decay, rot.

Depraved appetite: A desire for unnatural articles of food.

Differentiate: To establish a difference between.

Digestion: The process of converting food into materials fit to be absorbed.

Dissolve: To cause a substance to melt away in a liquid.

Docile: Easy to manage, gentle.

Dock: The solid part of the tail; also the parts around the anus.

Elbow: The bony projection at the upper part of the forearm

Excrement: The natural discharges of the body—feces and urine.

Excretion: The discharge of waste matter from the body, or the material so discharged.

Febrile: Pertaining to fever.

Feces: The discharges from the bowel.

Fetid: Giving off a bad odor.

Fetlock: The joint between the cannon and the long pastern bones. Also the lock of hair which grows behind this joint.

Fever: Abnormally high temperature of the body.

Fever, shipping: A general term applied to strangles, influenza, and contagious pneumonia occuring during or shortly after shipment.

Fistula: A long narrow canal caused by diseased action.

Flank: The soft part of the body which lies between the last rib and the point of the hip. It is bounded by the loins above and the belly below.

Flatulent: Distended with gas.

Forearm: The part of the foreleg between the elbow and the knee.

Forehand: The part of the horse in front of the saddle or rider. It includes the head, neck, and fore limbs.

Forehead: The upper part of the face.

Forelock: That part of the mane which hangs down over the face.

Function: The power of acting.

Fungus: A low form of vegetable life, as molds.

Gaskin: The part of the leg situated between the thigh and the hock.

Gastric: Pertaining to the stomach.

Gastritis: Inflammation of the stomach.

Germ: Any microscopic form of life.

Girth: The measure around the body at the chest.

Granulations: Small fleshy masses formed in wounds.

Hamstring: The great tendon which attaches itself to the point of the hock.

Haunch: The point of the hip.

Height of a horse: The distance from the ground to the highest point of the withers.

Hemorrhage: Bleeding.

Hock: The joint immediately below the gaskin.

Hypodermic: Under the skin.

Inaccessible: Out of the way.

Inclement: Harsh, severe; as weather.

Immunity: Security against any particular disease.

Indolent: Inactive. causing little pain.

Infection· The communication of disease from one animal to another.

Infectious: Liable to be communicated by infection.

Interdental: Situated between the teeth.

Intolerable: That which can not be endured.

Itch: An irritation of the skin with a desire to scratch.

Jugular: Pertaining to the neck.

Jugular channel: The groove which is on either side of the neck just above the windpipe.

Knee: The joint between the forearm and the cannon

Lamina (laminae, plural)· A thin, flat plate.

Laminar: Pertaining to the laminae.

Lateral: Pertaining to the side.

Lesion: Any change in the part of the body resulting from disease or injury.

Local. Restricted to one part.

Lumbar: Pertaining to the loin.

Massage: A stroking and kneading of the body.

Maxilla: A jawbone.

Maxillary: Pertaining to the jaws.

Membrane: A thin layer of tissue which covers a surface.

Microbe: A microscopic organism.

Microscopic: Visible only by the aid of a microscope.

Molar: Grinding; pertaining to the molar teeth.

Mortality: The death rate.

Muzzle: The lower part of the head, including the nostrils, lips, and chin.

Navicular: Boat-shapped, shuttle-shaped

Nodules: Little lumps.

Nonfebrile: Without fever.

Nourish: To furnish material to sustain life

Nucha: The back of the neck.

Odor: Scent, smell.

Ointment: A fatty medicinal preparation for external use.

Opacity: That which is opaque

Opaque: Having no luster; dull; impervious to light, not transparent.

Ophthalmia: Inflammation of the eye

Orbit: The bony socket which contains the eye

Organ: Any part of the body performing a definite function, as the liver, stomach, kidney, etc.

Organism: An individual animal, plant, or germ.

Ossification: The formation of bone.

Oxygen: A gaseous element of the air.

Parasite: A plant or animal which lives upon or within another plant or animal.

Parotid region: The region below the ear and back of the jaw.

Pastern: The region between the fetlock and the hoof.

Phalanx: A bone of the foot.

Phenol: Carbolic acid.

Pigment: Any coloring matter of the body.

Plantar: Pertaining to the sole of the foot.

Poll: The top of the neck immediately behind the ears.

Posterior: Situated behind or toward the rear.

Process: A projecting point.

Pulmonary: Pertaining to the lungs.

Pungent: Sharp or biting.

Pus: The creamy looking fluid resulting from suppuration.

Putrefaction: Rot, decomposition.

Pyramidal: Shaped like a pyramid.

Rectal: Pertaining to the rectum.

Retention; The keeping within the body of matter normally excreted.

Rump: The hinder parts.

Saliva: The fluid secreted by the glands in the mouth; spittle.

Sand cracks: Same as quarter cracks.

Scurf: Dandruff; a branny substance on the skin.

Serum: The liquid part of the blood.

Sheath: A double fold of skin which contains the penis.

Shoulder: That part of the fore limb which occupies the side and front region of the chest

Sinus: A cavity or hollow space, as of bone.

Skull: The bony framework of the head.

Shipping fever: A general term applied to strangles, influenza, and contagious pneumonia occurring during or shortly after shipment.

Slough: A mass of dead tissue in or cast out of the body.

Solution: A liquid containing dissolved matter.

Spine. A slender process of bone

Stifle: The joint between the hip and the hock

Streptococcus: A germ.

Stupor: Partial or nearly complete unconsciousness.

Suppuration: The formation and discharge of pus.

Susceptible: Capable of being infected or influenced.

Suture: A surgical stitch or seam.

System: A set of organs which unite in a common function.

Swab: A small stick with a piece of cotton on the end; used in applying medicine to wounds or sores.

Temperament: Individual peculiarity of physical and mental constitution.

Thoracic: Pertaining to the chest or thorax

Trachea: Windpipe.

Tract: A region, principally one of some length, as the digestive tract.

Transit: A journey from one place to another.

Transmit: To transfer; to pass on to another.

Transparent: Permitting the passage of the rays of light; clear.

Trunk: The body considered apart from the head and limbs.

Trypanosoma: A low form of animal life found in the blood of animals. It is the cause of surra and other similar diseases.

Ulcer: An open sore other than a wound.

Ulceration: The formation of an open sore.

Underline: The lower boundary of the chest and belly.

Vascular: Pertaining to or full of blood vessels.

Venous: Pertaining to the veins.

Vertebra (vertebrae, plural): Any one of the bones of the spinal column.

Villus (villi, plural): A minute projection from the mucous membrane of the intestine.

Vital: Essential to life; necessary

Vitreous: Glasslike.

Withers: The highest point between the shoulder blades.

INDEX.

216 INDEX.

www.ingramcontent.com/pod-product-compliance
Lightning Source LLC
Chambersburg PA
CBHW010043090426
42734CB00017B/3235